THE
ULTIMATE
GUIDE TO
BRACES

DR. BILL MARTIN

THE ULTIMATE GUIDE TO BRACES

A PARENT'S GUIDE TO THE NEW ORTHODONTICS

Advantage®

Published by Advantage, Charleston, South Carolina.
Member of Advantage Media Group.

ADVANTAGE is a registered trademark, and the Advantage colophon is a trademark of Advantage Media Group, Inc.

Printed in the United States of America.

10 9 8 7 6 5 4 3 2 1

ISBN: 978-1-59932-933-8
LCCN: 2018933440

Cover design by Carly Blake.
Layout design by Megan Elger.

This publication is designed to provide accurate and authoritative information in regard to the subject matter covered. It is sold with the understanding that the publisher is not engaged in rendering legal, accounting, or other professional services. If legal advice or other expert assistance is required, the services of a competent professional person should be sought.

Advantage Media Group is proud to be a part of the Tree Neutral® program. Tree Neutral offsets the number of trees consumed in the production and printing of this book by taking proactive steps such as planting trees in direct proportion to the number of trees used to print books. To learn more about Tree Neutral, please visit **www.treeneutral.com**.

Advantage Media Group is a publisher of business, self-improvement, and professional development books. We help entrepreneurs, business leaders, and professionals share their Stories, Passion, and Knowledge to help others Learn & Grow. Do you have a manuscript or book idea that you would like us to consider for publishing? Please visit **advantagefamily.com** or call **1.866.775.1696**.

TABLE OF CONTENTS

FOREWORD: FROM THE FOUNDER OF MARTIN ORTHODONTICS AND MARTIN KIDS DENTAL HEALTH TEAM. xi

CHAPTER ONE: WHY IS MY CHILD'S SMILE SO IMPORTANT?. 1

CHAPTER TWO: WHY DO KIDS NEED BRACES?. 9

CHAPTER THREE: WHY NOT JUST A DENTIST? WHY AN ORTHODONTIST? 15

CHAPTER FOUR: CHOOSE A HIGHLY SUCCESSFUL ORTHODONTIST 23

CHAPTER FIVE: WHAT CAN I EXPECT AT THE INITIAL CONSULTATION AND EXAM? 35

CHAPTER SIX: SHOULDN'T THERE BE A GUARANTEE? 41

CHAPTER SEVEN: HOW TO GET MORE INFORMATION 45

CHAPTER EIGHT: HOW TO PAY FOR ORTHODONTIC TREATMENT AND BRACES 49

CHAPTER NINE: AIRWAY ORTHODONTICS & YOUR CHILD'S PEAK PERFORMANCE 61

CHAPTER TEN: WHAT ARE THE TREATMENT OPTIONS? 77

CHAPTER ELEVEN: HOW DIFFICULT IS LIVING WITH BRACES 89

CHAPTER TWELVE: LIFE AFTER BRACES: RETAINERS 99

CHAPTER THIRTEEN: LET'S CELEBRATE! 103

CHAPTER FOURTEEN: WHAT ABOUT MY SMILE? 107

FAQ 111

RESOURCES 121

ABOUT THE AUTHOR 123

THE NEXT STEP: YOUR CUSTOMIZED SMILE ANALYSIS 127

Foreword

From the Founder of Martin Orthodontics and Martin Kids Dental Health Team

MY NAME IS DR. BILL MARTIN. I'm an orthodontist and the founder of Martin Orthodontics and Martin Kids Dental Health Team. My reasons for becoming an orthodontist and forming an organization committed to improving the health of kids—instead of becoming a Hollywood actor or a sports superstar—are simple: I want to change the world by helping kids be peak performers.

But this book is about *you,* the parent, and your son or daughter, not about me. It's about information you need to know to make intelligent, responsible decisions about your child's health, appearance, self-esteem, and social interactions ... of a permanent, lifelong nature. Does your child really *need* braces? If so, when? If so, who should you trust to provide his orthodontic care? How will you know you're not being ripped off?

This book isn't *Fifty Shades of Gray*. It just can't be that exciting. But if you take the time to read this book, you'll know how to confidently and correctly make whatever decisions you need to make about your child's orthodontic care.

It's *not* 1982.

To start, we're no longer dealing with heavy, ugly, tight, painful metal braces—every visit to have them tightened was another round of torture; they were hard to put on, hard to keep on, painful to remove, and it was irritating having a list of foods and activities to avoid for a long period of time. If your child needs braces now, the experience won't be anything like it was when you were a kid. He won't even try hiding under the bed and have to be dragged kicking and screaming to the car to visit my office.

Not only has *everything* about braces changed, but now all braces are created differently. So try to get that horrible, metal-mouth image out of your head. You're probably aware of invisible braces, maybe by a brand name: Invisalign. That's what prompts a lot of patients to call or email me in the first place. However, Invisalign is but one of a number of options to be considered to get to *the* best, customized, and personalized answer to your child's needs. You don't want to equate this to buying something over the counter: "Hey, give me Invisalign. How much?" It's more complicated than that. But it's a good representation of modern braces. They can be (nearly) invisible, pliable and with lighter steel, safer, and even self-removable for hygiene or sports and easily put back in place. They're not painful and achieve more certain results in a shorter period of time.

When I was growing up, a lot of kids didn't get braces they really needed and their parents let them off the hook, either because they believed their child couldn't tolerate the pain or because the cost was just beyond the family's budget. Now that braces are virtually painless, what about the cost?

Today's far better braces cost *less* than the one-size-damn-well-will-fit-all, metal-mouth braces of the '60s, '70s, and '80s. They cost as little as one Starbucks drink a day for a year, rarely more than twice that, and there are a number of different payment plans available if needed. So, that second hurdle is a lot lower than it was when our parents encountered it.

In other words, the first of my two introductory messages is: *relax.*

I've got your back. It's going to be okay—better than okay, easier than okay, and more convenient than okay. Orthodontic procedures *won't* hurt your child, and he or she will surprise you by not complaining it does. It's *not* going to hurt your bank account; you won't be reduced to a backyard stay-cation next summer and the summer after that. It's *not* going to be a maddening maelstrom of appointments of uncertain length, or hours in a waiting room: no emergencies from broken wires and loose braces, almost no time out of school or away from work. Not at *my* office.

More Than Just Braces

My second introductory message is: this is about more than just braces.

Orthodontic care for a child, preteen, or teen is more than just correcting crooked, crowded teeth with braces. That's like thinking diabetes only needs attention when feet have to be amputated, or getting tires checked might be a good idea after being stranded with a flat at night while it's pouring rain.

"Thank you for making our experience with braces pleasant and happy. As a busy working mom, I never knew it would be this easy and affordable."

—MARTHA, T.

Orthodontic checkups *by an orthodontist*[1], starting at age four of five, are a proper part of child rearing. In many cases, prevention is less troublesome and less costly. Even if you're late getting your son or daughter in, it's still possible they won't need braces and that other treatment options will do. But if they do need braces, the sooner you know of the options, the better.

This is also about more than just braces because it impacts psychological and emotional health, not just oral health. This is discussed later in the book.

Why It's Important

Individuals with an attractive smile may be judged as being more compassionate, more educated, more intelligent and more successful. It isn't fair, but facts are facts. First impressions can be made in just a few seconds, and if you're able to smile with confidence, you'll be able to make that first impression stick way better than if you were to hide a crooked smile. In addition, crooked teeth can affect your health in the following ways:

1. Straight teeth function better, are easier to clean, and are more likely to last a lifetime.

2. People with straight, well-aligned teeth can avoid gum disease, which has very serious health ramifications.

3. Properly aligned jaws reduce the risk of temporomandibular joint disorders (TMJ), which can ruin sleep or cause chronic headaches or migraines.

---

1   All orthodontists are dentists, but dentists are *not* the same as or suitable substitutes for orthodontists. Read on to find out more.

4. Crooked teeth are often a symptom of a much more severe health problem.

Some parents put off orthodontic treatment, but these irregularities and problems do *not* heal themselves. *This isn't acne; they don't grow out of it.* The problems only grow worse and harder to resolve with age.

Don't Ask Them to Hide Their Smile

Never smiling isn't easy in an age of selfies and social media. Children can become self-conscious—painfully self-conscious—and embarrassed. "No thanks, Mom, I'd rather just stay home."

Teen suicide has skyrocketed since social media shaming and bullying rose to ugly prominence. Teen depression affects everything from getting the good grades needed to get into a good college to first dates, first loves, and enjoying (or hating) their childhood and teen years. But it doesn't stop there. Uncorrected, bad smiles go with them to college and into their career.

This isn't just cosmetic either. It's also medical and can be a serious detriment to their health.

So, read on. Be informed. Be able to ask smart questions and do the right thing. I guarantee you'll be much better able to correctly and confidently make good choices for your family through this book.

Bill Martin, DMD

Founder, Martin Orthodontics and Martin Kids Dental Health Team

Chapter One

Why Is My Child's Smile So Important?

IF YOU ARE WEIGHING the yes/no and now/later decisions of orthodontic care or braces, you'll be trying to decide just how important or unimportant it really is.

Some parents feel "looks aren't everything." Some think their kid should just be tough-minded about this and not overly sensitive. Some may not have had orthodontic care when they were children and think, *Hey, I turned out just fine. I have a great spouse, a good career, friends—so what's the big deal?*

But that was then. This is *now*: the age of social media.

Social shaming and bullying is a lot worse, a lot more common, and a lot more persistent than when you were a kid. Teen suicide is on the rise, and such suicides share one thing in common: shocked and bewildered parents who could not conceive of their child ending his own life. Sure, they might've noticed he was a *little* depressed. They knew he was being bullied and spending more time home, alone, not leaving his room, but geez, he *is* a teenager, after all. What once was a few days or weeks of misery contained in the cafeteria with a few bullies is now endless, expansive, and broadcast online to everybody. Behind a computer screen, it can get far nastier than most would dare in person. Sometimes, kids bully each other for no reason, being a buck-toothed girl or a boy with gaps in between their teeth is enough to exacerbate the situation.

Signs Your Child May Be Being Bullied

- decrease in self-esteem
- not wanting to go to school
- skipping school
- injuries they can't explain
- self-destructive behaviors (e.g., harming themselves)
- declining school grades
- sleep difficulties
- loss of interest in schoolwork or activities
- sudden loss of friends or avoiding social groups
- changes in eating habits

A straight, clean and healthy smile can not only give your child the confidence she needs to embrace her true worth, but can also pave the way toward easier socialization at school, church, or during extracurricular activities. Do your child a favor and talk about her smile and how it might be affecting her.

Beyond that, there's a life ahead of your child. Going to junior high with crooked teeth and a humiliating smile is one thing. Hey, plenty of kids are going to school *without shoes* for heaven's sake. But going to college admission interviews, packing up and heading off to college, going to job interviews, trying to fit into new and anxiety-rich environments at a faraway college or new workplace with a bad smile—and maybe unavoidable bad breath with it—and daytime headaches from nighttime teeth-grinding is a lot more serious.

This isn't *just* a cosmetic issue. Misaligned, crooked teeth equal *significant* medical problems.

Poorly aligned teeth can produce chronic headaches and migraines, contribute to digestive problems because of the inability to properly chew foods, and make getting a decent night's sleep impossible. Perhaps the most dangerous of all: it can foster gum disease. Gum disease has absolute links to diabetes, heart disease, strokes and dementia, as well as, of course, the loss of natural teeth altogether. Orthodontic corrections later in adult life are more difficult; they can be painful, require time off work, and at best, they'll just be embarrassing. *Invisible braces aren't really totally invisible, and you're thirty-eight? Forty-four? Fifty-one? C'mon.*

Uncorrected mouth problems and misaligned teeth make for strangely stretched gums inevitably destined to separate from teeth. This could allow "pockets" for infections and periodontal disease to arise and turn into *very* difficult, painful, and costly problems late in life.

In the teenage years, failure to spend even $4,000 can easily create a $40,000 full mouth restoration case at age forty or fifty, or embarrassing, health-compromising removal of all teeth and use of dentures at age sixty.

Gum disease is serious business. It worsens the risks of and heightens dangers from diabetes, heart disease, strokes, and dementia. Ignoring preteen or teen teeth misalignment may virtually guarantee adult medical problems. If there is a genetic history of any of these medical problems I just named, you only worsen the odds of your son or daughter suffering from them by ignoring or postponing needed orthodontic treatment.

Aside from impacting health, a poorly aligned smile can significantly impact your child's comfort. Headaches, toothaches, sinus problems, dry mouth, snoring, drooling, bad breath, and insomnia are all symptoms of a smile that isn't straight, jaws that aren't aligned, or teeth that are too close together or not quite close enough. Oftentimes, however, the mouth is the last place we check for signs of discomfort, loss of sleep, or even a simple headache.

If your child's pediatrician can't figure out why she's not sleeping well or experiencing headaches or even insomnia for which there seems to be no cause, a simple thirty-minute exam at your local orthodontist could provide a clear solution in no time!

Here is what I'm told by an awful lot of parents:

> "I had wonderful parents, *but* I sure wish they had found
> a way to afford the braces I needed and gotten me the care
> I needed when I was a kid, so I didn't grow up to have this
> bad smile my whole life."

And what I hear from almost every adult patient getting orthodontic treatment and braces is:

> "I had wonderful parents, *but* I sure wish they had found
> a way to afford the braces I needed and gotten me the care

I needed when I was a kid, so I didn't grow up to have this bad smile my whole life *and have all these problems now.*"

Is this how you want your daughter or son talking about you ten, twenty, or thirty years from now? Is this how you want them remembering their childhood? Your parenting?

If that sounds pretty damned pushy, I admit: it is. I kept it in the book for the very simple reason that this is *truly* what I have heard so much over the years, and I am sincere about letting you reflect on it. All parents want to do the right thing. They don't want to let their children down in any way, and I'm sure you don't either.

You know, parents just about kill themselves over their kids' college, trying their best to guide the decision, trekking around the country on campus visits, worrying over campus culture, or taking on *serious* debt. Every parent understands what many kids can't— that it's not about the few years of college but rather the forty or fifty years afterward.

I assure you, this is the same. It's not about the bad, humiliating smile and bad bite transformed now, for high school. It's about the many, many years to come. They really can't appreciate that now, but *you* can.

No parent wants their child to suffer, either from teeth that actually hurt, headaches you can't explain, insomnia that affects their daily life, or insecurity your child may be feeling because of a crooked or oversized smile. The fact is, your child's formative years are actually the most sensitive for his or her teeth. Now is the time to pay close attention to your child's smile, behavior, peer relationships, and confidence level.

If any or all are lacking, a qualified orthodontist may help give you and your child the peace of mind you both crave.

The Top Five Reasons People Avoid Seeing the Orthodontist

1. **Patients are afraid it's going to hurt.** Pain is the number-one reason most people avoid going to the orthodontist. However, modern technology—and choosing the right orthodontist—can ensure that your child enjoys a pain-free orthodontic experience.

2. **Patients are afraid it's going to cost too much.** Not only are most orthodontic procedures more afford-able than ever, but insurance, payment plans, and a variety of other financing options make this all but a moot point for most of my patients. Remember, orthodontists aren't in this to get rich, they're here to make sure your child's teeth, smile, and jaw are aligned to make his or her life better—period! We're not going to let something like price get in the way of creating a better, safer, healthier smile for your child.

3. **Patients are afraid it's going to take too long / they're going to miss too much school or work.** Regardless of the type of orthodontic procedure your child needs, time is of the essence. Modern technol-ogy and ease of access allows us to work around your child's school schedule with minimal absences. After initial visits, and barring the actual procedure

itself, most visits and/or adjustments are routine and can take anywhere from fifteen to forty-five minutes.

4. **Patients do not see the need to take action.** Eroding, crooked, or unaligned smiles can take time to happen, but the time to act is now. Orthodontic irregularities don't just heal on their own or disappear if you ignore them. Your child's smile and overall dental health are too important to ignore out of questions of pain, convenience, or even price.

5. **Patients have been treated in the past with an attitude of indifference.** Let's face it, not all doctors are created equal. Every profession has its "bad apples," and to say dentistry is the exception would be to write fiction instead of fact. There is no room for indifference when it comes to your child's healthcare. Find an orthodontic specialist that offers not only state of the art technology for your child, but state of the art service as well. Orthodontic specialists know what it's like to sit in the chair, and should provide every opportunity for patients, especially our younger patients, to feel comfortable, safe, and secure in our care.

Call us at **352-371-3200** or go to **MartinKidsDental.com** to schedule your own Customized Smile Analysis.

Chapter Two

Why Do Kids Need Braces?

ARE BRACES SOMETHING CREATED by orthodontists to make money, like Disney and their extra-charge FastPass? Was it a conspiracy from the very start?

Then and now, there may be some overprescribing and premature prescribing by some doctors. There are bad apples in every orchard. And you know the adage: if all he's got is a hammer, everything (and everybody) looks like a nail.

But there is a very legitimate, clinically documented, and 90 percent of the time, clearly visible reason why some kids, as young as eight, *need* orthodontic treatment and care: malocclusion.

Malocclusion is a fancy-pants term for all things related to misaligned teeth—teeth growing angled, crooked, and into a too-crowded space. It can be a single tooth, a few teeth, or the whole mouth. As I said, it is partly hereditary, and your kids didn't get to pick their parents out of a Barbie catalog. There can be other causes too, like poor breathing, poor oral habits such as thumb sucking and mouth breathing, and premature loss of primary teeth.

If your child is suffering from any, several, or all of the following early indicators of malocclusion, consider having them addressed by an orthodontic specialist sooner rather than later:

- **Mouth Breathing:** If I had to pick one thing that I see cause malocclusion more than other causes, it would be mouth breathing, instead of breathing through the nose. This may also be caused due to a stuffy nose or enlarged tonsils and adenoids. If you can't breathe through your nose, the upper jaw will not grow properly and there will not be enough room for the teeth to come in straight.

- **Crossbites**: A crossbite occurs when the jaw deviates to one side with an improper fit of the upper and lower teeth from left to right or front to back. Crossbites can lead to worn and chipped teeth, jaw pain, and asymmetric growth of the jaws. Left untreated, the crossbite will require more extensive treatment later in life and significant jaw surgery in the most-severe cases.

- **Poor Oral Habits**: Thumb-sucking habits, poor swallowing, and tongue thrusting should be corrected immediately in order to prevent severe jaw and tooth alignment problems.

- **Miscellaneous concerns**: There are several associated issues you should also be looking for as soon as your child turns seven in order to intervene early, including the following:

  □ permanent teeth that are growing into the wrong spots

- severely protruded front teeth at risk for injury or causing teasing at school
- severe crowding with permanent teeth erupting into poor-quality gum tissue

With any of these situations, we can discuss the pros and cons of early intervention and treatment versus waiting until all the permanent teeth are in for braces. If you are anxious about the appearance of your child's teeth or your child is self-conscious about his or her appearance, early treatment might be the best choice. Not only are most orthodontic problems more difficult to correct later, but self-image and personality inhibition can be hard for a person to leave behind. However, if your child is extremely resistant to treatment or is not mature enough to be trusted to care for their teeth, delay may be the better choice. In that case, regularly scheduled orthodontic checkups will be necessary.

Having malocclusion does *not* guarantee a child will need braces. Frankly, this is what worries me about nonspecialists like family dentists substituting themselves for orthodontists, and parents letting it happen. They may easily miss an early diagnosis of malocclusion, when it could have been treated without braces. Or they may leap to braces as the only way to treat all malocclusion. Either way, you and your child lose.

The first question, then, is: does your daughter or son have or show all the signs they are going to have malocclusion? Second, if so, what—of numerous options—should be done about it? Third, when?

To have all these questions answered early, the first full orthodontic exam should occur early in a child's life. That is why I started

Martin Kids Dental, so a children's dentist trained in recognizing problems with the way a child's mouth is developing can alert the orthodontist for early intervention. We like to see kids when the first tooth comes in, that way many of the problems we see at eight or nine can be prevented.With early and periodic exams by an orthodontic specialist, you may avoid your child's need for braces and/ or you may prevent years of suffering and embarrassment related to their teeth and smile.

Waiting will have very serious consequences, often requiring more treatment and higher costs later in life. What most parents fail to realize is that these treatment problems are urgent and should be treated as such. If that ship has sailed, the next best time for a full orthodontic exam is tomorrow at three o'clock.

If your son or daughter does need braces—now or at some predictable future time—the outcome of the exam can lead to *sensible* decisions. If not now, treatment to prevent the need can begin, and also, you can begin saving money for braces or other procedures if necessary later on in your child's life. There is no tooth fairy coming to leave a few thousand dollars underneath his pillow or yours. But if the need must be met three years from now, skipping one Starbucks run a week for those three years can make a hefty dent in the bill to come. Utilizing a Health Savings Account or Flex Spending Account can help, as well. How to fund orthodontic treatment is discussed later in the book.

Let me be emphatically clear. I am *not* in the business of putting braces on any child who doesn't need braces. My office is *not* a braces store. I'm in the business of helping kids and families get the right orthodontic treatment if any is needed, get the right braces if any are needed, and have as perfect a smile and as few oral health problems as possible. I make sure my patients are informed—that's why I wrote this book. In my office, you're never told what to do. You're provided with real information, no medical jargon, plain English, "reasons why," and options. You probably know the term "God complex," referring to a person who acts like he's God—imperious, brusque, and deliberately intimidating to squash questions. You will *not* get that kind of treatment here, from me or anyone on my team.

Kids do need braces, but not all kids and certainly not the same braces for all. Some kids are better served by other orthodontic treatments instead of or before braces. We will collaborate, you and I, to figure out what is or isn't needed and what options are best if there is a need for your child.

Call us at **352-371-3200** or go to **MartinKidsDental.com** to schedule your own Customized Smile Analysis.

Chapter Three

Why Not Just a Dentist?
Why an Orthodontist?

YOU UNDOUBTEDLY ALREADY have a dentist.

Gee, isn't seeing an orthodontist going to cost a lot more?

I'm busy. More appointments?

Do I really need to get orthodontic checkups for my kids?

Don't worry, these are all reasonable questions! It is true that, today, quite a few dentists dance over into our territory, and although they're *not* permitted to claim they're the same as orthodontists or provide orthodontic treatment (beware of any who do), they're able to do things like provide Invisalign and other braces. This can be confusing. Here are the facts.

All orthodontists are dentists and we all graduate from the same dental schools. True enough. But that's where it stops for dentists. Orthodontists go to school for an additional two to three years to become credentialed specialists at diagnosing and providing the best treatment for conditions like:

- mouth breathing
- difficulties chewing or biting
- constant biting into the cheek, gums, or roof of the mouth
- teeth that meet abnormally or don't meet at all
- teeth grinding or clenching
- crowded, misplaced, or blocked out teeth
- early or late loss of teeth
- teeth grown in badly
- teeth that protrude
- embarrassing personal appearance due to teeth
- facial imbalances
- teeth or jaw misalignment, TMJ
- chronic headaches and migraine
- poor sleep
- speech difficulties (that may never be outgrown or may develop later)

These are *not* dental care issues. They are orthodontic issues.

For *some* things, a generalist or jack-of-all-trades will do. For other things, you know it's smart to seek out the best specialist you can afford. For example, if all your income is in a single W-2 from one employer and you have simple, ordinary deductions, getting your taxes prepared for the cheapest fee at the seasonal H&R Block office that opens up in your neighborhood shopping center is probably fine. But if you have W-2, 1099, and investment income from real estate, depreciation on real estate in several states, own stocks, and you raise iguanas as a money hobby, you're going to get yourself a really good accountant, probably a CPA. If you need the simplest will, leaving everything first to spouse or second to daughter may be okay. But if you are of some means and have several children and maybe also grandchildren as well as charities, you're going to need to see an *estate planning* attorney, not just any attorney—though they all went to the same law schools—but *a specialist in estate planning.*

This is no different.

There are a few things to keep in mind when differentiating between a general dentist and an orthodontic specialist.

First, generalists, or jacks-of-all-trades, tend to work with one-size-fits-all, off-the-rack, standardized solutions. They may be limited to doing only what the computer dictates that they do, without bringing expertise and expert judgment to bear. They're often working with products from only one provider, without being able to select from a full range of options that would work best for you. Specialists, instead, tend to individually and carefully diagnose needs and provide personalized solutions.

Second, generalists and their use of inexpertly applied, standardized solutions tend to be cheaper than the fees of a specialist, but that also places economic pressure on them to do the treatment as quickly and simply as possible, because they've "cut it thin."

In this case, it's worth remembering that the treatment provided has permanent, lifelong, and life-impacting consequences. This concerns your health, future dental or jaw alignment or misalignment issues affecting quality of sleep (which can affect weight, even onset and management of type 2 diabetes and heart disease), as well as self-esteem and social and career success.

> **General Dentist.** A general dentist gives routine checkups, preventative measures, cleans teeth, and fixes cavities. They may not start seeing children until they are seven to ten years old.
>
> **Children's Dentist.** A children's dentist just sees children and adolescents. They have specifically studied the needs of kids in order to have an understanding of what is needed to have a healthy adult mouth. They provide dental care to children and adolescents, and offer checkups, preventative measures, cleanings, and treat cavities.
>
> **Orthodontist.** An orthodontist has two to three years of specialized education beyond dental school and is an expert at straightening teeth and aligning the jaws. They assess patients and determine the best treatment routes and procedures that need to be taken.

If you can, you want to choose an orthodontist for orthodontic care.

You may ask, *how do I know my doctor is an orthodontist?* It's a good question and a critical one to ask as you seek additional treatment for your child's dental issues.

Only orthodontists can belong to the American Association of Orthodontists (AAO). If you're looking for a local orthodontist, go online and visit **www.braces.org** to find a specialist in your area. This website features not only a searchable database of orthodontists but educational tips, answers and resources to help you on your quest for your child's healthiest smile!

Alternatively, you can ask your doctor if he or she has completed a two- to three-year residency in orthodontics and check with your state dental board to follow up on his reply. Dentists and orthodontists in most states will be registered differently with the dental board.

Do your homework; be a "dental detective" while on the hunt for such vital information. Look for the words "dental specialist in orthodontics," or ask your general dentist for a referral to a specialist. In urban and suburban areas, it will take minimal effort to find a specialist. In more remote, rural locations, your search might take you to another city or town. Don't be afraid to ask your dentist if an orthodontist travels to your town every month to see patients. There's a chance an orthodontist from a larger city comes to your town and works out of another dental office once or twice per month. Looking around can save valuable driving time and money.

One note: there is no disrespect between orthodontists and dentists. As a matter of fact, many orthodontic patients are referred by their dentists. These are great, capable, and caring professionals who know where their expertise begins and ends, and who do not let ego or income opportunity step in front of what they know is best for their patients. Just as the family doctor refers his patients with possible or significant heart disease issues to a cardiologist, and if need be, the cardiologist refers to a surgeon, the best dentists refer patients with orthodontic needs to orthodontists. Orthodontists are required to take two to three years of university education beyond dental school and additional continuing clinical education every year. They must also invest in state-of-the-art technology for their offices (not found in dental offices)—*all for a good reason.*

Even though we orthodontists have the education and training to perform general dentist procedures, we don't. We specialize.

> Call us at **352-371-3200** or go to **MartinKidsDental.com** to schedule your own Customized Smile Analysis.

Chapter Four

Choose a Highly Successful Orthodontist

WHY IS THAT IMPORTANT? Wouldn't you get a "better deal" from one barely getting the light bill paid? Maybe. But an overeager orthodontist—or maybe more so, an overeager dentist eager to do braces—might be seeing needs that are more urgent than they really are.

What are some good clues to selecting a great orthodontist?

I've got two: his practice is busy.

I assure you, the ability of advertising to attract orthodontic patients is limited and it's expensive. When you see a really, really busy practice, there are probably a whole lot of patient referrals, and neither kids nor parents enthusiastically refer if they feel they were lied to or treated badly, put in pain, or wound up with results nothing like the digital future-photo they were shown. And they probably wouldn't come to that practice if they had to keep coming back to "fix a few things," or were overcharged. Parents tell parents about great orthodontic practices because we earned their trust and because their kids keep thanking them.

I keep my office very busy. Yes, we advertise. But mostly, these practices thrive by patient referrals. Not that I would anyway, but I don't need to goad you into more and more expensive care than your son's or daughter's situation requires for the best outcome. I don't need to "sell" four more sets of braces this month to win a cruise from the manufacturer—and yes, that stuff goes on in some practices. There's an old cartoon from the *Wall Street Journal* with a bunch of executives in a boardroom at a conference table, one hollering, "Ethics? Ethics? We can't afford ethics!"

This is a business, a business built on ethics and earned trust. And you do *not* just need a doctor to install braces; you need a trust-worthy advisor.

The other clue: a great orthodontist is *not* cheap.

Our fees are calculated to allow for "Cadillac + Care" in every respect, to put no downward financial pressure on how we care for patients and parents, and to *never* cut corners or take shortcuts. We *never* use any material that is "probably good enough."

If I were you, I'd worry if I could find an orthodontist that is a lot cheaper than anywhere else. If you do find one, know this: behind closed doors they're probably asking, "Can we do this cheaper?" Is *that* the question you want discussed back there, at every step of your child's treatment?

This isn't even like Botox. It's more like cosmetic surgery. There's a science and an art to this. My team and I are all highly trained to produce state-of-the-art outcomes, nothing less. The doctor makes a difference. That's why I tell everybody to get a highly successful orthodontist.

The Top Ten Things You Should Know *Before* Choosing Your Orthodontist

This is something you want to be sure about.

I've just suggested one big consideration: a very successful practice. Here are ten more.

1. Are they a specialist?

Orthodontists are specially trained dentists who take on several extra years of training in order to "straighten teeth," usually by affixing braces to the patient's teeth. You might say we specialize in smiles. Orthodontists also perform dentofacial orthopedics. This is a fancy way to describe how we normalize the structure of a patient's jawbones in order to repair any imbalance in their face. All orthodontists are dentists, but only 6 percent of dentists are orthodontists. Look for the seal of the American Association of Orthodontists (AAO). Only orthodontic specialists can belong to the AAO.

2. Do they treat adults?

Orthodontics is not just for kids! It's important that your orthodontist can treat patients of all ages. Many adults are finding out how a healthy and attractive smile is important to their health and the way they feel about themselves. Others choose to avoid a lifetime of crooked teeth for health concerns or problems with their bite.

3. Do they provide the first visit free of charge?

Most orthodontists offer free examinations for new patients so you and your family can get expert advice about treatment needs, options, and timing before making this important investment. During your first exam and consultation be sure your questions are answered, your concerns are addressed, and you are educated about all of your treatment options. The orthodontist should include digital x-rays during the exam at no charge.

4. Do they offer guarantees? If so, what are they?

No matter which orthodontist you choose, ultimately you are not making a small investment. That being said, wouldn't you want to ensure your orthodontist is going to stand behind their treatment? Of course! We wouldn't have it any other way. In fact, we offer a satisfaction guarantee. If your child has any issues or if you are not satisfied with the treatment, our team of smile specialists will make it right, guaranteed.

5. Are they using the latest technology and treatment options available?

Orthodontics today differs a great deal from years past. 3-D x-ray imaging lets us diagnose "why" you have malocclusion at half the radiation of conventional x-rays. Computer-designed braces and wires dramatically increase the precision with which we move teeth and shorten treatment time. Clear braces offer a cosmetically pleasing alternative, while Invisalign/Clear Aligners offers patients an entirely brace-free option. Did you know that Invisalign also has a special treatment system just for teens?

Ultimately, you get the best treatment available when you choose us.

6. Does their quoted fee include retainers?

Each orthodontic office has its own fee schedules, and doctors often charge differently for procedures. All orthodontists should offer you a contract that clearly spells out the expenses for your child's treatment before it begins.

Throughout the orthodontic industry, it's common to find out about retainer fees after you start treatment. You should ask your orthodontist about what retainers cost and also if there are any other hidden fees.

7. Do they charge for emergency appointments?

Some minor discomfort may occur with braces. Orthodontists typically provide adjustments for poking wires and loose appliances free of charge. While we do provide these types of adjustments free of charge, you should definitely ask about adjustments and potential costs with your orthodontist before you start treatment.

Keep in mind that if your braces are broken or damaged due to noncompliance with dietary restrictions, this may result in repair charges. If you do your best to avoid breaking your braces and follow the simple dietary guidelines that we will share with you, then you should have no additional costs for adjustments throughout your treatment, even if it's an emergency.

8. Do they make you feel special and comfortable?

Regardless if you are reading this book for your own treatment or for your child's treatment, when you meet with your orthodontist, you should definitely feel comfortable. We strive to make you as comfortable as possible before, during, and after treatment. You are special and we want you to feel special every time you see us.

Particularly important if you are reading this book for the treatment of your child, we also ensure your child feels special every time they visit. Since our doctors are so involved with children and young adults, we can empathize, relate to them, and make them feel comfortable and extra special.

9. Do they have a great reputation?

With the internet, it is extremely easy to pull up ratings and reviews from patients. Simply go to Google and search for orthodontist reviews and ratings in your town.

Additionally, look on the website for video testimonials from actual patients. You can also ask the orthodontist for references.

Finally, you should make sure your orthodontist is a member of the Better Business Bureau and has a great rating with them. Being a member of the BBB shows you that the orthodontist takes pride in providing great customer service and treats patients the way they should be treated.

10. Are they flexible with payment options?

Once you are comfortable and you know specifically which orthodontist you want to treat you or your child, the next question is typically, "How much is this going to cost and how am I going to pay for this?"

We help you understand different payment options from maximizing the most insurance benefits to flex spending accounts to even interest-free payment plans. During the initial exam and complimentary consultation, we will answer all of your questions, including those about our typical cost of braces and the variety of payment options available.

How to Know What Questions to Ask

I've really thought through the questions most parents and patients have—not just the ones they ask, but the ones they don't. This book attempts to cover them all, but again, this is a *personal* matter. The best questions to ask are the ones that matter most to you and your child.

I hope not, but you may be in a position that absolutely requires you to get the minimum essential treatment for the lowest cost. If so, your most important questions are going to be about those kinds of options and about price, and nothing else.

If, however, you are able to make your decision about who you should trust with your child's oral health and smile by many factors, we've included a "What Is Most Important to You?" quiz on the following pages. As you'll see, there are fourteen different items to consider and rank in importance to you. Any can become the questions you ask me and my team or any other orthodontist.

If you have a specific question not answered anywhere in this book, or have a personal and confidential question, you can—with complete assurance of privacy and courtesy—email us at smile@ martinkidsdental.com or call and ask for the Orthodontic Treatment Coordinator at 352-371-3200.

There is also a FAQ section at the back of this book.

Of course, a perfect opportunity to get questions answered— yours and your son's or daughter's—is at your exam appointment.

Call us at **352-371-3200** or go to **MartinKidsDental.com** to schedule your own Customized Smile Analysis.

What Is Most Important to You?

Directions: For each **Key Item** below, rank its importance to you from 1 to 5. Then check off whether each type of provider provides that item. When you're done with all 14 Key Items, add up your rankings and review what your final score means about choosing an orthodontist.

	Key Items to Consider in Selecting Your Orthodontist	Rank How Important Each Item Is to You in Selecting Your Orthodontist 1 – Not Important, 5 – Very Important	Martin Kids Dental	Other Provider	Other Provider
1	Orthodontist and staff committed to expert, thorough diagnosis, and prescription of the best treatment plan customized for my son or daughter	1 2 3 4 5	✔		
2	Avoiding extractions (if possible)	1 2 3 4 5	✔		
3	Avoiding having to wear headgear with braces (if possible)	1 2 3 4 5	✔		
4	Avoiding "metal-mouth" braces (if possible) or utilizing the new type of "invisible" braces	1 2 3 4 5	✔		
5	Having a healthy, pleasing smile that will last a lifetime and protect optimum dental health (not just having straightened teeth)	1 2 3 4 5	✔		
6	Pain-free treatment	1 2 3 4 5	✔		
7	Orthodontist utilizes the most modern, advanced, and proven technology, including computer-aided design and fitting	1 2 3 4 5	✔		
8	Orthodontists and team actively involved in continuing clinical education	1 2 3 4 5	✔		
9	Reducing treatment time to a minimum without compromising results (including total length of treatment term and number of office visits)	1 2 3 4 5	✔		
10	Availability of after-school or after-work appointment options	1 2 3 4 5	✔		
11	Treatment coordinator is knowledgeable about insurance coverage and is able to offer flexible payment plans	1 2 3 4 5	✔		

12	Getting the best overall value factoring in thorough diagnosis, customized care, and concern with lifetime health and well-being—not just the cheapest fee	1	2	3	4	5	✓		
13	Lifetime guarantee	1	2	3	4	5	✓		
14	Orthodontist and team committed to excellence in orthodontics and customer service for both patients and parents	1	2	3	4	5	✓		

Total of Your Rankings

What Your Score Means

50-70 There is no doubt. Martin Kids Dental is the right choice for you and your family! It is clear that you place a high value on a comprehensive, "best" approach.

43-49 You are probably also going to be happiest with Martin Kids Dental, rather than any other alternative. But this score suggests you aren't completely sure and have some unanswered questions or concerns. Your doctor and the practice's treatment coordinator want no lingering uncertainties on your part, and want to address any and every question. Don't keep anything to yourself. Please ask.

42 or less Frankly, you may not value the advanced, sophisticated level of clinical care and customer service provided at Martin Kids Dental. Cost may be much more important to you than other factors, or very basic service may be all you feel you need. It's perfectly okay. If you choose to shop around, be sure to use this checklist in evaluating other options. Remember, you do want everything right the first time, and you want error-free orthodontics at a minimum.

Chapter Five

What Can I Expect at the Initial Consultation and Exam?

MANY QUESTIONS SURROUND YOUR first visit to a new orthodontist, not the least of which is the subject of this particular chapter: *what will happen at the initial consultation?*

To answer this very common question, and perhaps several others you might not even realize you need answering yet, let me walk you through the typical first office visit, from the initial appointment forward. Your first appointment is scheduled following your initial phone call to your orthodontist's office.

1. **On arrival at the office, you will be greeted by one of our certified treatment coordinators**. She or he is fully prepared to make everything from the first appointment to an entire treatment program go smoothly for you and your child. Your treatment coordinator will manage your relationship with us, from appointment scheduling for your convenience to answering questions.

At the initial visit, your treatment coordinator will review your child's patient information and health history and/or any appearance concerns with you.

This interview and required-by-law paperwork doesn't take long. You may also be asked to view, with your son or daughter, a pre-exam video.

2. **Next, your orthodontist will conduct the "Customized Smile Analysis,"** the most complete and thorough orthodontic exam, including teeth, gums, mouth, jaws, and face. Typically, safe digital x-rays are taken of the teeth and surrounding bone and of the jaw structures.

Usually that same day, your orthodontist will present his or her "report of findings"—a "show-n-tell," in plain English (not medical jargon), of the full state of your child's teeth, gums, mouth and jaws, and a diagnosis of any present or anticipated problems that should get orthodontic treatment. If treatment should occur, your orthodontist will present recommendations and options. This will be an individualized, personalized plan of treatment, not "braces in a box, off the shelf." By this report of findings, you will know:

- what teeth or jaw misalignment or other problems exist or are developing

- what the health and appearance ramifications are of not intervening with treatment

- if braces are needed now or later and which type of braces will be best in your situation

- what the complete treatment program will consist of, such as braces, number of appointments, and average time of each office visit

- what results will be achieved at the end of treatment

3. **All your questions will be answered**. There are no dumb or embarrassing questions. Every single one of my patients has a question, simple or complex! We do *not* want you or your son or daughter just nodding, then later wondering, "What did he mean by *that?*" or saying, "I wish I'd asked about ..." This is *not* one of those "I'm the doctor—trust me—just do what I say because I said so" offices. So, any and all questions you have should be asked and answered. Our goal is not just a terrific orthodontic outcome ensuring a healthy, attractive smile, but also your anxiety-free comfort from start to finish.

4. **Finally, your treatment coordinator will explain the costs of the prescribed treatment program and discuss payment arrangements as needed**. Before proceeding, the next two appointments will be scheduled for the installation of braces and/or other treatment. As the saying goes, a journey of a thousand steps begins with the first one, and a task well begun is sooner done!

In total, you should allow about one hour for this entire initial consultation and exam.

If that seems like a lot, keep in mind there are *lifetime* health, appearance, and personality aspects of this. And it's not "installing tires"—not if it's done properly and expertly. Your son or daughter deserves a careful, thorough, and anxieties-eliminated experience. You want to make the best decisions for them.

Frankly, our practice and our process is not for everybody. We attract and "resonate with" parents who are quite serious about their responsibilities and committed to giving their child every possible advantage in life—certainly not unnecessary disadvantages. If you are that parent—and the fact that you took the trouble to obtain and read this book suggests it—then you are going to recognize that this is time well invested in the best possible results.

Call us at **352-371-3200** or go to **MartinKidsDental.com** to schedule your own Customized Smile Analysis.

"Our experience with the orthodontist has been better than we ever expected. My son is so proud of his smile, more and more every day."

—MARY C.

Chapter Six

Shouldn't There Be a Guarantee?

HEALTH CARE IS NOTORIOUS for no guarantees.

Surgeons have a dark-humor insiders' joke: dead patients can't sue.

If you've seen reality TV shows about plastic surgery, like the popular one airing as I wrote this, *Botched*, you know things can go horribly wrong.

Guarantees are controversial in all kinds of health care, including orthodontics. Many doctors are upset by the very idea. One huffed and puffed at me, "What do you think you're doing with this guarantee nonsense? We aren't operating a car shop, installing mufflers and guaranteeing them for five thousand miles. We are doctors, dammit."

His ego was mightily offended. But I doubt you will be, with the challenge of deciding who should be your family's *trusted* orthodontist. So, yes, I think there should be a guarantee! In fact, many guarantees!

1. **If you aren't satisfied with your son or daughter's orthodontic treatment, new smile outcome, or patient/parent experience, *our team of specialists will make it right, guaranteed.***

2. **Also, the quality of the orthodontic treatment itself is *guaranteed for life*.** If ever the proper teeth alignment originally achieved somehow begins to fail, we will welcome you back and do everything we can to correct the problem.

3. **You also have a safety in numbers guarantee.** The diagnostic and prescriptive methods and state-of-the-art technology and the braces products we use have been used by top orthodontists nationwide to treat over one million patients successfully.

4. **You also have my guarantee that *every* orthodontist and orthodontic assistant at my office has been not only academically educated but also *thoroughly* trained.** They all follow the same proven method to diagnose needs, plan the best and personalized treatments for every patient, and manage for best results from day one through after-care. There is nobody "learning on the job" with your child—ever. All patient care is supervised and reviewed by me. We also invest in frequent state-of-art clinical continuing education for our team exceeding all state licensing requirements. Above and beyond.

5. You also have ***my guarantee of exceptional courtesy and customer service***. Yes, you are my patient, but

we can be honest about this—my practice is not just a health care provider, it is a *business*. As such, it has, in my opinion, one set of responsibilities to you as the parent of a patient and one set to the patient, including telling the whole truth and nothing but the truth, prescribing in the patient's best interest, and delivering the best possible treatment and outcomes. There's also a second, separate set of responsibilities to you as a customer, including access, convenience, responsiveness, and "red carpet service."

These five guarantees are included in your treatment program fee.

For starters, I can guarantee you the best, most thorough orthodontic exam, and I encourage coming in for it now.

Call us at **352-371-3200** or go to **MartinKidsDental.com** to schedule your own Customized Smile Analysis.

Chapter Seven

How to Get More Information

THERE ARE SEVERAL WAYS to get information about an orthodontic practice. First, I want to address the ways I don't recommend.

I don't recommend Yelp. Yelp is, unfortunately, not at all what it seems, and is frequently the subject of lawsuits from business owners, under regulatory scrutiny centered around the poorly policed manipulation of reviews, and has even been accused of the flooding of fake reviews—by "bots" no less! Some companies can use Yelp as competitive warfare while other companies turn around and sell the business owner under negative-review-assault "reputation management services." So, beware! Get the information you need from truly trusted sources.

Google can also be deceptive, though I admit it can be a valuable starting point. Rankings are manipulated by advertisements, websites, YouTube content, and what's called SEO, or search engine optimization. The only thing you know for sure about dentists or orthodontists who come up at the top in Google rankings in your community is that they are good at SEO or, more likely, good at paying somebody who is good at SEO. They're willing to spend money and willing to create a lot of content. Does that equate to certainty of the best diagnostic expertise, treatment, patient care, and customer service? Sometimes. Sometimes not.

So, first, the best thing to do is make certain you get all your questions answered by the orthodontist and the practice's treatment coordinator. Don't hold back. Put them on the spot. Be assertive. Don't feel you have to be deferential to the doctor! My own goal in this is to have every patient and every patient's parent *fully* knowledgeable about every aspect of the treatment so that they have *zero* anxiety.

Second, if you have a quick follow-up visit scheduled, these are wonderful opportunities to either ask questions you may have missed the first time, or to get further details from your orthodontist directly.

Now that we know where to get your most burning orthodontic questions answered, here are some simple tips I've amassed over the years to help you easily and effectively get the information you need:

How to Get Your Questions Answered

Make a list. The easiest way to get what you want is to know it in advance. Make a list of the various questions you have when they arise so you can quickly and easily go down the list to assure you've got the right answers for the right questions.

Bring it with you. Take the list with you when you go for your child's orthodontist visit. This way you have the questions at hand at the right place at the right time. If you're calling in to get answers, you can also have the list ready and tick off one question for every answer you receive.

Record the answers. If your orthodontist, or their receptionist, speaks too fast or you can't keep up while writing the answers down, why not record them? Your cell phone likely has a "record" feature, and if not, there are many affordable micro-recorders on the market today.

Double-check. Finally, make sure you have the right answer by double-checking with your orthodontist or their receptionist or assistant.

Knowing where to find the information you need is only half the battle; follow these tips and you'll know how to get what you're looking for as well.

Regardless of how many questions you have, or your comfort level with technology, phone calls, or in-person visits, your orthodontist should offer an option that fits your schedule and makes all your unresolved issues crystal clear.

Call us at **352-371-3200** or go to **MartinKidsDental.com** to schedule your own Customized Smile Analysis.

Chapter Eight

How to Pay For Orthodontic Treatment and Braces

YOU MAY HAVE NEVER needed braces. Or you may have needed them and gotten them. Or you may be among the tens of thousands of people in our generation who needed them but did not get them, perhaps because your family decided they couldn't afford them. Maybe they didn't consider it a priority and probably underestimated the lifelong results of the decision. You may not only have lived with a "hide your smile" habit unnecessarily, but you may have developed chronic jaw pain and headaches, difficulty chewing, or even periodontal disease that could have been prevented.

Regardless of which group you're in—and I hope it's not the third—I hope you will be making the best choices for your son or daughter today, without being hamstrung just by the finances. Truth is, parents pay out the same cost for a number of different things not nearly as vital as health or emotional well-being without blinking, mostly because it's paid in installments or just never really *considered*, like the monthly cost for minutes/data on mobile devices, added up for a year or two. The additional insurance cost and other costs when the teenager gets his driver's permit; after all, what's the choice? The cost of braces leaps up and stands there, all at one time. So, it can seem big. And it tempts thoughts of, "maybe later," or, "is this really necessary?"

I hope in the prior chapters I have succeeded at getting the "is it really necessary?" question erased. If there is a visible need or if expert examination by an orthodontist and his explanation of what he finds shows you it's necessary—then *it is* necessary! It won't fix itself. It will probably get worse. It plagues a person's health, emotional well-being, social life, and career. It can link to very serious medical problems. *Necessary* is not really debatable.

Now let's tackle the ugly matter of the money.

I say "ugly" because nobody really likes talking about this. Most orthodontists are nervous about it. Parents are uncomfortable with it. If there is a financial obstacle to treatment, most people are reluctant to admit it, offer other excuses, and then can't be helped by the doctor. I think we have to trust each other. With me, this discussion is entirely confidential, in a "safe zone." Orthodontists are not Martians, by the way; *we* have kids, college tuitions that loom, and family budgets.

What Is a Reasonable Fee and Cost?

A complete treatment program, including braces, can cost anywhere from $4,000 to $10,000 or so. Most fall in between. Adjusted for inflation, these prices are actually *less than* braces decades ago, while the technology and quality has advanced. In costs it can prevent later, it's a bona fide bargain. TMJ treatments are expensive. Cosmetic dentistry work is expensive. Migraine headache drugs are expensive and have side effects.

For this investment, you will be getting the carefully selected, personalized solution to your child's irregularities and problems, prescribed using state-of-the-art digital technology along with the expertise of a specialist, and considerate, compassionate care from start to finish. Your investment includes a varying number of appointments plus the orthodontic appliance itself, after-care, and in my office, certain guarantees.

It's hard to really draw a fair comparison, but if you have any significant net worth, you can easily pay similar fees for the services of an attorney expert in estate planning. Most kitchen remodels cost considerably more. Where real expertise is involved and the stakes of getting it wrong are high, you can't escape professional level fees.

In this case, the $4,000 to $10,000 range is seen as perfectly reasonable by the overwhelming majority of parents that I talk to. Each year, we provide braces of one kind or another to countless patients. Even parents who shook their heads at the cost to start with tell me afterward that having witnessed everything we do to get the absolute best obtainable results, and seeing the outcome itself, they feel undercharged.

While it's never easy to part with such a sum, people do it every day for all sorts of less important things, like their new designer handbag, golf vacation, or suite of living room furniture. They'll pay for it outright or with their favorite credit card (getting the reward points in the bargain). If you put the orthodontic treatment program including braces on a typical credit card at the interest in play as I write this, and you choose to make only the minimum required monthly payment, your monthly payments will be relatively small.

Even tight budgets can accommodate this *when it is really important.* It's less than most families pay for their cable and streaming entertainment. For many, if they got all their Starbucks stops consolidated into one monthly bill, it would be more than this!

Health Spending Accounts (HSA) / Flex Spending Accounts (FSA)

The HSA allows you to set aside *pre-tax* dollars to be used for certain medical and health expenses for you or your family. They exist although restricted under the Affordable Care Act (Obamacare) as it stood in July of 2017. By the time you read this, the opportunity may have been expanded, as President Trump suggested. In any case, if you have accumulated money in an HSA, you can probably spend it on orthodontic treatment. If you don't have an HSA, you might want to start one. Information can be found online about existing or new accounts and their rules of use, at www.healthcare.gov.

Other kinds of FSAs are typically set up through your place of employment and similarly enable you to set aside pre-tax dollars for medical expenses. Sometimes, employers match contributions. Again, you can almost certainly tap funds from your FSA for your child's orthodontic care. Check with your employer about this.

If you have a tax accountant, you may want to consult with him about your HSA or FSA.

TIP: How can you make the most out of your employer's flex-pay plan? First, make sure you understand how it works. Second, set aside flex-spending dollars in advance of need, and if possible, make the maximum contributions. Many employers allow higher limits than you'd think without asking, as much as $2,500 to $5,000 per year. Be aware of "family status changes" allowed by your plan that may enable you to change the amount being moved pre-tax from your paychecks to your account anytime during the year rather than just once at the first of the year—so you could bump up the amount in months before the first orthodontic treatment. IMPORTANT: be aware of the balance and the loss of unused funds. In most cases, if you do not use these funds, you lose them, year to year. You usually have three months after the end of the calendar year to submit claims for eligible expenses from the previous year.

Insurance

These days, there are as many different types of insurance plans as there are patients in my office. I can't possibly speak to your unique and personal insurance policy without seeing it first but, in general, my experience tells me that "most" insurance policies cover "some" of your orthodontic expenses.

I realize that answer sounds very vague, but here are a couple of variables you need to answer before an insurance agent can help you determine what, how long, and how many procedures fall under your insurance:

- the type of procedure (braces, Invisalign, etc.)

- the duration of the procedure (two months, six months, a year, etc.)

- the cause of the procedure (a patient presenting with pain, a parent's concern, traumatic injury or accident, congenital birth defect like cleft lip or palate, etc.)

- the nature of the procedure (to correct pain/discomfort, cosmetic, etc.)

I can only partially answer this question, but talking to your insurance agent will help you get the right answers you need.

TIP: Keep an insurance journal of every interaction with your carrier. Write down the date, time of call, name of the person you contacted, and the exact instructions or recommendations following the call. Later, if your insurance company doesn't remember what they told you, you'll have it accurately written down. If they still don't remember, ask them to pull the recorded audio tape from your previous call, so that you can accurately "remind" them of exactly what they told you.

Loans

Most orthodontic offices offer a couple of payment plans, but if they don't fit your budget, you are usually out of luck. Luckily, we have partnered with a company OrthoFi. With OrthoFi, we can allow you to fully customize a payment plan to match your budget, so you never have to sacrifice quality treatment for financial reasons. You don't need to go anywhere else to apply or do paperwork; we can take care of it in my office.

If you have equity in your home, the lowest-cost loan option may be a home equity line of credit or second mortgage. See your own bank, or check out RocketMortgage at rocket.quickenloans. com. As of this writing, mortgage interest is at record lows.

Obviously, a private loan from a family member can be the easiest option. A lot of preteens' and teens' important orthodontic care is financed at the Bank of Grandma and Grandpa.

What If You Really, Really Can't Afford Braces?

I have compiled a list of eighteen ways you may be able to substantially reduce the cost of braces. Frankly, some of them are less than ideal, and most are not available through my office, but they could be helpful if your back is really up against a financial wall.

1. **Get braces in April or November and see if you can save a little extra by paying in full.** These are the months that orthodontists are the least busy, and it's when we have our most meetings (April–May). In November, everyone is getting ready for the holidays or the office is closed the week of Thanksgiving. By scheduling during the "off season," you can often find better deals with willing orthodontists.

2. **See if you can get a discount for not breaking any brackets.** Believe it or not, most orthodontists would happily take $100 off your final bill if you don't break any appliances throughout treatment!

3. **New technology; better pricing.** See if you can be one of your orthodontist's first patients with a new technology and save some money on the lab fee or receive a discount for being a teaching case.

4. **See if your local dental school has an orthodontic program.** The treatment at such institutions is supervised by orthodontists. While you will spend a little more time in the chair as a teaching case, if you have the time, it might be well worth the wait because you can save up to *half the cost of traditional braces.*

5. **Ask your insurance plans when they send out their fee schedules to participating providers.** If the insurance company updates their fees or the orthodontist raises his or her fees to keep up with the cost of inflation, it might be around November in preparation for the next year.

6. **See your dentist every four to six months.** While you're wearing your braces, the extra cleaning each year can prevent tooth decay, a costly item to repair.

7. **Get your flex spending dollars in order with your employer.** If you set money aside in a flex plan, it may be "tax-free," but it comes with some stipulations: namely, you have to use it before the end of the year or else you lose it.

8. **See if you can get a second set of retainers from your orthodontist at the end of treatment.** Sometimes getting two sets of retainers at the same time can be cheaper than buying a second set later in life when you lose or break your first set.

9. **See if your husband or wife has an insurance plan that covers braces.** Be sure to enroll in the plan with enough time to spare before your child needs braces, so that the procedure is not denied by your insurance company due to a waiting period.

10. **Ask for flexible financing options.** When you boil it down to the basics, your orthodontist really just wants to help you. Regardless of his specialty, your doctor spent way too much time in school *not* to love what he does. If you're easy to work with, keep your teeth clean, and avoid breaking your braces while you're wearing them, he or she will probably be thrilled to help you finance the care, or find another way to afford the investment.

11. **Do you have multiple kids in treatment?** If so, take advantage of that fact and see if you can get a family discount.

12. **If finances are extremely tight, you should check out the organizations that orthodontists have created to help provide pro-bono care, such as Smiles Change Lives.**

13. **School auctions, churches, or public service entities will often receive donations from local orthodontists wishing to donate a case to the school or organization for a fundraiser.** Checking around local school newsletters or church bulletins for their upcoming silent auctions could be a great find! If you're unwilling to leave such things to chance, call your local schools or churches and ask them specifically if they have such a fund and, if so, how to apply/qualify.

14. **If you're thinking about a career change, apply at your local orthodontist's office.** Most orthodontists offer free braces to their staff and their children as an employee benefit! (And you never know, you could love your career *and* your child's new braces!)

15. **Military personnel, schoolteachers, and firefighters sometimes receive special courtesies in dental and orthodontic offices throughout the year.** Keep your ears open and you might save a few bucks or at least get a donation from the orthodontist to your organization.

16. **This tactic won't save you any money, but it could earn your organization or business some money if you have a newsletter, sports team, fund-raiser, or special event that needs a sponsor.** Ask your orthodontist. Most orthodontic offices are huge supporters of the communities in which they practice and would probably love to advertise with your organization.

17. **Got taxes?** Good! Why not use your tax refund to help pay for treatment in full and ask for a courtesy on the average fees associated with financing a full orthodontic case? In some areas, you can save as much as 10 percent on the cost of braces by simply saving your pennies and paying the entire bill at once, up front.

18. **Ask for more flexible financing through a third-party credit company like Chase Healthcare Advance, CareCredit, OrthoFi, or by using in-house financing through your orthodontist.** Most orthodontists will accept a reasonable down payment and split the remaining amount into easy monthly payments for your convenience.

With automated withdrawals from a checking or savings account, you might be able to stretch the monthly payments out over a longer period to make each payment lower. Just don't be shocked if your orthodontist asks you to approve a credit check. A little homework up front can be well worth the effort when your monthly orthodontic bill is lower than your cell phone bill!

There's no doubt about it; this investment in your child's future can be expensive, but your return on investment will be far better than any other. However, now that you're armed with these eighteen massive, budget-saving tips, you won't need to decide between braces and your budget ever again!

Call us at **352-371-3200** or go to **MartinKidsDental.com** to schedule your own Customized Smile Analysis.

Chapter Nine

Airway Orthodontics & Your Child's Peak Performance

AIRWAY ORTHODONTICS, AS the name suggests, is about breathing. You need oxygen to survive, which is why your body makes breathing its number-one priority—even more important than hunger or thirst. However, the way your body receives oxygen can be surprisingly complicated.

To help you understand airway orthodontics, I want you to think of a light switch. When the switch is on, the light turns on. When the switch is off, the light turns off. Most people think of breathing the same way. Either you have oxygen, or you don't. The reality, however, is much more complex.

The truth is, breathing works more like a dimmer switch. When the dimmer switch is at full brightness, you have full light. But a dimmer switch can also be partially turned down, so the light may only be a glimmer. Oxygen works the same way. Your body may only get a trickle of oxygen at times. It's enough to keep you alive, but it's not the full amount needed for optimal health.

What Are the Effects of Low Oxygen on Your Child?

When your child can't breathe well, their body senses the problem and reacts with stress. This causes your child to adjust their behavior subconsciously to improve the flow of air. One common adjustment is to start breathing through the mouth instead of the nose, especially if the nose is swollen inside or blocked. Your child may do this because they are trying to reduce the stress on their body by getting more oxygen.

The long-term effects of mouth breathing and other resulting behaviors are terrible and often ignored. These issues can stretch into adulthood and include:

- Sleep deprivation and fatigue

- Heart disease

- Depression

- Arthritis

- Anxiety

- Muscle aches and spasms

- Poor posture and resulting spinal pain

- Rapid aging

- Obesity and weight problems

- 20 percent shorter life expectancy

- Increased risk of numerous illnesses, including cancer, diabetes, Alzheimer's disease, and dementia

Most of these effects won't show up until your child becomes an adult, but there are also negative effects that can appear during childhood. Unfortunately, these effects are frequently misinterpreted as symptoms of another ailment or even ignored as temporary behaviors that a child will outgrow with time. In truth, however, these symptoms can serve as early red flags that there is a problem with your child's breathing.

Does Your Child Suffer from Any of These Symptoms?

The following can be symptoms (and in some cases, the cause) of lowered oxygen levels in your child:

- Bedwetting
- ADD / ADHD
- Poor memory
- Social difficulties / problems making or keeping friends
- Low energy
- Allergies
- Negative thoughts / pessimism
- Excessive temper tantrums
- Snoring, heavy breathing, and/or open mouth while sleeping

- Sleepwalking or night terrors

- Open mouth or slack mouth when awake

- Chronic earaches

- Dental issues, such as crooked teeth or increased tooth decay

- Headaches in the morning

- Dark circles under the eyes

How Are All These Problems Related to Breathing?

For many of the symptoms listed here, poor nighttime breathing is the ultimate culprit. The fact is, when you're asleep, your body is on autopilot. It shuts down systems such as your voluntary muscles. In this way, the energy you usually use to move your body around gets redirected to take care of other critical functions. While you're asleep, your body clears out the waste that builds up in your cells during the daytime, and your brain also uses extra energy to process everything you experienced when you were awake.

You can compare sleep to the neighborhood garbage truck. You and your family create trash each day in your home. Empty milk cartons. Broken toys. Vacuumed dirt and debris. Used paper towels. The filth builds up, and you put it into your trash can. You bring your trash to the street, and the garbage truck hauls it away.

But what happens if that garbage truck never comes? What happens to your house then?

Your home will turn into a dumping ground. The filth will build and build. You'll never be able to mop the floors, because the garbage will be in the way. You'll never be able to bring in new things, because the old, broken trash will take up all the space in your house. You won't be able to keep up with maintenance, and your house will start to look like something out of *The Addams Family*.

Sleep is your body's garbage truck. If you don't get enough of it, your body cannot clear out its waste. When that happens, all sorts of systems can begin to go haywire.

This brings us back full circle to the list of symptoms in the previous section. It is during sleep that children grow and develop the most. When your child doesn't get enough sleep, growth gets interrupted—emotional growth, cognitive growth, and physical growth. And one of the biggest culprits for poor sleep is—you guessed it—poor breathing.

Connecting the Dots

Sleep consists of four different stages: falling asleep, light sleep, deep sleep, and REM (dreaming) sleep. You start in one stage and then cycle back and forth through the other stages throughout the night. Here is a brief review of those four sleep stages:

1. **Falling Asleep.** This is the "nodding off" stage. You may still have mild awareness of your surroundings, but you are transitioning into an unconscious state.

2. **Light Sleep.** Now you are asleep. Your brain and muscle activity begin to slow down, but they are still working to

some degree. Your heart beats more slowly. Your body's temperature cools down.

3. **Deep Sleep**. Your brain and muscle activity have slowed significantly. Your muscles go into extreme relaxation, which saves your body's energy for other processes. This stage of sleep helps injuries heal. It also restores physical energy to your body.

4. **REM Sleep, aka Dreaming Sleep**. About sixty to ninety minutes after falling asleep, you begin to dream. During this time, your muscles are paralyzed, but your brain is extremely active. It processes experiences from the day and creates long-term memories. In children, this stage is critical for emotional and intellectual growth.

Each stage of sleep allows your body to grow, heal, and process in different ways, and each stage is critically important to you and your child's overall health.

For children who suffer from poor breathing and low oxygen, however, their body's autopilot forces them to wake repeatedly throughout the night. The first stage of sleep—light sleep—typically proceeds without much issue. When a child enters deep sleep, however, the relaxation of the muscles causes a collapse of the airway. This makes it even more difficult to move air in and out of the lungs. The child's body doesn't get the oxygen it needs, so it turns on its stress alarm. The alarm forces the body to return to the former "light" stage of sleep, allowing the airway to reopen. Because of this, the child never finishes a deep sleep cycle, and they possibly never even start the critical REM dreaming stage.

To summarize, poor nighttime breathing habits can stop healthy sleep from happening. Without healthy sleep, a child cannot develop their optimal physical, emotional, or intellectual health.

This is where airway orthodontics enters the picture.

How Can Orthodontics Help Your Child's Breathing Problem?

To answer this question, I want to share two patients' story with you. For privacy, I will call these patients Mary and Robbie.

Today, if you met Mary, you'd know she is an intelligent, beautiful young girl who is thriving in school. Her rounded face has a healthy sun-kissed glow to it, and her smile naturally reaches the outer corners of her sparkling brown eyes.

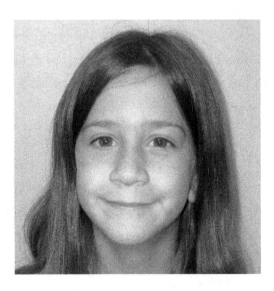

Now let me introduce you to Mary one year ago. Mary's mom brought her to me when she was five, because she was worried about crooked teeth. I quickly recognized that these teeth were only one symptom out of many others.

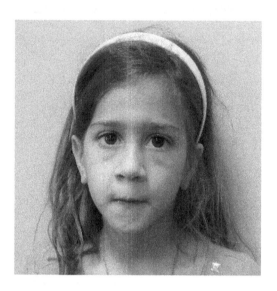

When I first met Mary, my eyes weren't immediately drawn to her striking eyes and smile. The first things I saw were dark, bruised-looking patches of skin that sagged under her tired eyes. The second thing I spotted was her mouth—not a smile, but rather a thin set of tightly pursed lips that were barely wider than her nose. She drew her eyebrows together when she looked at me with an expression of tension and worry. The child was clearly exhausted.

I wasn't the first person to notice that Mary was suffering, of course. Her mother knew, but she was at a total loss for what to do. Mary's pediatrician had written off her appearance and tiredness as the unavoidable side effect of "allergies." Lucky for Mary, she had a smart mother who knew something had to be done and who wouldn't rest until her daughter was taken care of.

Mary's diagnostic imaging came back to show an airway that was horribly constricted. Her so-called "unavoidable" allergies had resulted in enlarged tonsils and adenoids. Her upper and lower jaws were not growing sufficiently to accommodate her teeth and tongue. This left almost no room for air to pass easily into her lungs, especially during sleep. In addition, Mary's allergies forced her to breathe through her mouth instead of her nose. As a result, she wasn't holding her tongue or facial muscles correctly. She wasn't swallowing correctly. All of this caused her developmental problems to get even worse.

I referred Mary and her mother to a local ENT (ear, nose & throat doctor), who removed Mary's tonsils and adenoids. Once she had healed from that procedure, she returned to me for early orthodontic treatment. I fitted her with an orthodontic appliance that helped to guide her upper and lower jaws' natural growth. In this way, I widened her jaw to accommodate her teeth, tongue, and airway. She is now undergoing specialized physical therapy (known as myofunctional therapy), which is teaching her how to hold her tongue in the right position, swallow correctly, and breathe through her nose. As you can see for yourself in her current photograph, she is now experiencing some of the best sleep of her life.

The second patient story I would like to share is that of Robbie, who first walked into my office when he was seven years old. He was referred to us because he had a narrow upper jaw, a crossbite, and front teeth that were coming in "crooked and bucked out."

When I walked into the examination room, my eyes landed on a "wired" little boy who simply couldn't sit still. His tired appearance included dark circles under his eyes, and he was breathing with his mouth open.

Before I pointed out my immediate observations about Robbie, I first took the time to hear his mother's concerns. We talked about Robbie's crooked and protruding front teeth. Because of his appearance, Robbie was being teased in school by the other kids. Unfortunately, this is a frequent concern I hear from parents. Teasing and bullying can be a common experience for children who struggle with overtly crooked teeth.

After our initial conversation, I examined Robbie and reviewed a 3-D scan of his head and neck. I saw enlarged tonsils and adenoids, narrow upper and lower dental arches, severe crowding of the teeth—all of which led to mouth breathing. When Robbie's mom and I looked in his mouth, she commented that his tongue looked huge, like someone was "trying to park a Hummer into a Volkswagen parking spot." I explained that his tongue wasn't really large—the issue was that his jaws were too small. His tongue was being forced toward the back of his throat, making it hard for him to breathe whenever he was lying down.

Once I had pointed out the orthodontic problem, I then said, "Let's talk about *why* Robbie has crooked teeth that stick out." I had his mom fill out a Pediatric Sleep Questionnaire. (You can view this questionnaire yourself by visiting www.MartinKidsDental.com/Airway.)

The history that unfolded from the questionnaire was striking. Robbie was a heavy breather when he slept, and he rolled restlessly all over his bed. He always seemed to have a stuffy nose from allergies and frequent colds, and he often complained of having a sore throat. Allergy treatment had been unsuccessful, and the pediatrician had only said Robbie would eventually "grow out of it."

Meanwhile, Robbie's demeanor during the day appeared to contradict itself: he would somehow be both hyperactive and tired at the same time. He was failing in school but had tested gifted. His mom was sad because he didn't fit in at school with the other kids.

He struggled to keep friends because he was "constantly annoying them." When it came to sports, he was typically the last kid picked because he was notorious for getting out of breath too quickly. To compensate for his social struggles, he escaped into the world of computers and video games.

It broke his mother's heart to see Robbie struggle so much. With no better option available, she had agreed to put him on ADHD medication so he could survive at school. Still, she hated the idea that her son would be on medicine forever.

After hearing Robbie's history from his mom, I told her about the relationship between childhood breathing and sleep, and how the interaction between the two can affect the growth of a child's face and the development of their mind. If a child doesn't breathe well, then they don't sleep well. The subsequent sleep deprivation can lead to other physical and behavioral problems.

I sent Robbie to an ENT who also understands the important link between breathing and sleep (unfortunately, not all of them do). Robbie's tonsils and adenoids were removed, and he had a procedure done so he could finally breathe through his nose. Then, he returned to my office, where we expanded both jaws to create more room for his tongue and teeth. We started working with him to improve his diet, and we showed him how to correct the poor oral habits he had acquired to survive. He needed to "retrain" his tongue now that he could breathe better. We worked on breathing through his nose, tongue position, and proper swallowing.

After two years, Robbie is now a totally different kid. He sleeps well at night, can run and play sports without getting winded, is off his ADHD medication, makes better grades, and is easier to be around. As with any similar case, he didn't turn into a perfect kid overnight, but he continues to make improvements daily.

Stories like Mary's and Robbie's bring me joy, and reinforces my purpose: To be able to open a new door for a child, to illuminate the path toward a life of improved health and success—this is why I view airway orthodontics as one of the most important medical fields emerging today.

What Exactly Is Airway Orthodontics, Then?

To put it simply, airway orthodontics is a subsection of orthodontics that transforms children into peak performers. It does this by making sure they can breathe right, especially when they're asleep.

Orthodontic treatment may sometimes be the answer to a child's breathing problem, and sometimes another treatment from another type of doctor will be better. As in the case of Mary, she benefited from my orthodontic care, but she also required help from other specialists—an ENT and an allergist. The fact is, breathing and sleep incorporate numerous systems in our body. The reason for sleep disturbance in one child can be entirely different than in another child. Every case needs to be looked at as a unique, complex situation with a multi-part solution.

That's part of the problem, though. All of these specialists look at a patient through their own narrow view of medicine. They can't always see the forest through the trees. This is where airway orthodontics is unique. We are specialists, yes—specialists of the jaw and teeth—but we recognize the ways jaws and teeth relate to the rest of the body. We have trained beyond the scope of orthodontics, so we can recognize when other specialists should be called.

When Should Your Child See an Airway Orthodontist?

In an ideal world, every child would be evaluated at birth.

Now, that response may sound a bit tongue-in-cheek, but hear me out. Typically, orthodontics is a profession that treats deformities after they have already formed. Are your child's teeth crooked? Does the bite align correctly? Does your child have an overbite or underbite? These are some examples of problems that braces seek to treat after your child's jaw and teeth have finished developing. Early treatment seeks to head off some of these deformities before they have cemented in place, but even then, the problems have already become apparent. The teeth are already starting grow in crooked, or the jaw's growth has already been inhibited to some degree.

Airway orthodontics goes a step further than early treatment. It asks the question, "Why are these deformities happening in the first place? And what can we do to keep them from ever starting?"

The answer to this question will vary from child to child. To find the answer for your own child, the airway orthodontist looks at certain behaviors and factors that can affect the way your child's teeth and jaw grow. Consider this: From the day your child is born, their muscles are growing and becoming more coordinated. They slowly learn how to use their hands to grab and hold things. They eventually learn how to stand and walk with their legs. They learn how to make sounds with their mouth and tongue by moving muscles in certain patterns.

While all this learning and muscle training happens, a baby is also learning how to position their tongue in their mouth. They are learning how to swallow. They are subconsciously training themselves to breathe in a certain way. All of this will affect the subsequent physical development of a child's jaw and airway passage.

Yes, in an ideal world, every child should be evaluated at birth. That being said, what is a practical approach you can take in your world, right now?

First, I recommend you seek out a pediatrician who understands the important link between abnormal breathing during sleep and various medical symptoms and behavioral problems, or at least, a pediatrician who is willing to have a conversation about it.

Second, I recommend you bring your child to an airway orthodontics specialist by the age of four or five years old. The ages of five and six are critical for cognitive development, and losing sleep during this time can significantly impact your child. By having your child evaluated by a trained airway orthodontist, you can truly set them up for a lifetime of healthy development.

What if your child is already older than five? Don't worry! Even when I see patients at the "traditional" orthodontic age of twelve years old, I can still help them!

The fact is, there will always be options to improve your child's breathing and sleep at any age, from childhood into adulthood. Remember, though, that the sooner you start the path toward healthy breathing, the sooner your child can truly reach their full potential.

Do You Want to Know More?

To learn more about the science and benefits of airway orthodontics, visit **www.MartinKidsDental.com/Airway**. While there, you will be able to:

- hear additional stories of children who flourished after they regained their healthful sleep;

- watch videos explaining the science and biology behind airway orthodontics;

- take an Airway Assessment to see if your child demonstrates common symptoms related to sleep and breathing;

- contact Dr. Bill Martin and his team with any additional questions you may have about airway orthodontics and your child's health.

Call us at **352-371-3200** or go to **MartinKidsDental.com** to schedule your own Customized Smile Analysis.

Chapter Ten

What Are the Treatment Options?

IF YOUR CHILD IS ready for orthodontic care, one of the first discussions to have with your orthodontist is which procedure is right for him or her; there might be more options than you had ever imagined.

If you're like most people, you associate orthodontists with braces, but these days, that is just one arm of what I or any orthodontist does. Here are some of the services most orthodontists will provide their patients with during the course of routine treatment:

- metal braces

- Invisalign clear removable aligners

- clear braces

- expanders to match jaw size and tooth size

- space maintainers

- retainers to prevent crowding and shifting of teeth

- functional appliances to help improve facial balance

- early treatment and growth modification

- customized appliances designed uniquely for each patient

While many of these services may seem self-explanatory to you, several will probably not. In the following pages, I will try to elaborate on several of them, including:

- crossbite correction

- metal braces

- clear braces

- Invisalign

Crossbite Correction

As your child's teeth begin to grow in, there's a *lot* more at work than mere gum lines, tooth fairies, and molar size. How the jaw is shaped, when it develops, and even how "normally" it develops can all affect the placement and comfort of your child's teeth.

Most crossbites are the result of a narrow upper jaw due to poor nasal breathing which causes the upper teeth to bite inside the lower teeth.

Your child might have a crossbite if, for instance, the lower jaw is out of line with the upper jaw (kind of like a box that won't close right because one of the hinges is bent).

Or perhaps on the right side of your child's mouth, the lower teeth "stick out" a little farther than the top teeth, making the upper teeth on that side overlap in turn.

Or maybe your child's upper and lower jaws are out of alignment so instead of the top and bottom front teeth meeting "naturally" as they should, the front teeth fall somewhat behind the lower teeth. This would be the reverse of an overbite—you'll hear this referred to as an "underbite" or "anterior crossbite."

As you might imagine, any or all of these developments can lead to short- and long-term discomfort for your child.

How, When, and Why Crossbites Form

You might be amazed to find out how many ways a crossbite can form as your child grows and develops during his or her formative years. Heredity is one key to jaw growth, or alignment, as is the size of your child's developing jaw.

Another factor that can contribute to the development of a potential crossbite is if it takes your child too long to lose his or her baby teeth. In some extreme cases, in fact, if it takes too long for your child to lose his baby teeth, another set of teeth can grow in behind them, throwing the alignment off and contributing to a crossbite.

Believe it or not, something as basic as whether your child breathes through her nose or her mouth can also contribute to a crossbite. While most children breathe through their noses, some children develop a habit early on of breathing through their mouths instead.

In children who breathe through their noses while they're sleeping, the tongue naturally rests on the roof of the mouth, promoting natural and proper upper jaw growth. When young children breathe through their mouths, however, the tongue relocates from the roof of the mouth to the bottom, removing that extra support and potentially contributing to reduced upper jaw bone growth; this can create the crossbite we spoke of previously.

How Can I Spot a Crossbite?

Although it sounds severe, and even painful from the description provided earlier, the effects of a crossbite can take time to manifest themselves. Still, here are some of the telltale signs your child might be cultivating, or already suffering from, a crossbite:

- snoring

- difficulty breathing

- chewing on one side of the mouth or the other

- signs of an underbite

- if your child's chin seems "off center" or disproportionate

How, When, and Why to Correct a Crossbite

Where should you start looking for treatment if you're concerned about your child's jaw development after reading this section? If you suspect your child might have a crossbite, contact an orthodontic specialist and have your child evaluated.

There are many possible treatments available for a crossbite, and your orthodontist can work with you closely to make the right and specific decisions for you and your child.

When should you start? I believe you know my standard answer when it comes to questions like this one: *as early as possible*! The same way an auto mechanic would tell you to take care of that oil leak, bulging tire, or faulty timing belt sooner rather than later, myself and my colleagues in orthodontics will always favor early treatment to later.

Crossbites are often closely linked with other orthodontic issues, such as teeth alignment, jaw size, and growth, so naturally, the sooner you address any or all of these issues, the better.

Finally, why should you address a crossbite? Crossbites can lead to pain, discomfort, lack of space for the teeth to come into the mouth and a lack of confidence as your child begins to feel insecure or even ostracized because of this very treatable, very normal series of jaw and teeth developments. If your jaw has to shift to an abnormal position so your teeth can touch, it will grow in that position, resulting in an asymmetric face.

Not only can crossbites become physically uncomfortable if left untreated, but if the misalignment or root cause of the bite isn't fixed early in childhood, then the child's appearance and, ultimately, confidence could be affected as the crossbite becomes more pronounced in adolescence.

Types of Braces

There are basically two types of braces: metal and clear. There are many manufacturers of braces, and you may hear about Damon braces, Inovation braces, and more—with claims about faster and easier treatment. The bottom line is, the way a case progresses and finishes boils down to the skill and expertise of the orthodontist, not necessarily special braces. This is another reason you should choose an orthodontist to do your treatment versus a general dentist.

Metal Braces

The fact is, metal braces still have a valued place in the orthodontic world, and despite advances and breakthroughs of products like Invisalign and even clear braces, they aren't going extinct anytime soon! This is because metal braces are very strong and can withstand most types of treatment. Today's metal braces are smaller, sleeker, and more polished than ever before. Often the wire is attached to the braces with colored elastic ties. Kids have a blast picking different colors for their braces.

Clear Braces

Ceramic braces are very strong and generally do not stain. Adults like to choose ceramic because they "blend in" with the teeth and are less noticeable than metal. These are the type of braces actor Tom Cruise had.

Adult Orthodontics

It's not uncommon for individuals who have undergone orthodontic treatment earlier in life to find their teeth have drifted out of alignment over the years. Most adults won't think twice about bleaching their teeth to roll back the effects of time. Yet few think about the role orthodontics can play.

Adults of all ages can enjoy the same cosmetic and health benefits of properly aligned teeth with clear braces of Invisalign.

Improperly aligned teeth can do more than undermine your confidence. They can make proper cleaning and brushing more difficult, contribute to enamel loss, and even set the stage for more significant problems down the road. Fortunately, discrete treatment can help keep you aligned with a healthy, happy lifestyle.

The Solution Is Clear

Orthodontists believe every individual has the right to live their life with a smile they truly love, particularly children. Healthy, straight, and attractive smiles make your child happier and more self-confident. And isn't that what we all want for them?

"Our son has a lot of anxiety about visiting any doctor, but the transition into the orthodontics world was very easy and painless for our family. Thank you for all that you do to bring beautiful smiles to our family and many, many more!"

—MOLLY H.

Invisalign (Clear Aligners)

Invisalign is a widely advertised, well-known, and popular braces product, and kids often know about it and ask parents and doctors for it by name. Invisalign is a brand name for what is referred to as a Clear Aligner. Invisalign was the first company to make clear aligners, but there are several other manufacturers to choose from. Your orthodontist will know how to choose the best company for your individual situation. For many, it's as good an option as any other and sometimes even the best option.

Invisalign uses advanced, proprietary 3-D computer-imaging technology to "map" the entire span of treatment, from the present teeth alignment to the desired positioning, alignment, and smile. Clear aligners are custom made and based on the 3-D imaging. Invisalign has many features that have helped make it such a popular choice. The aligners are removable, even before a snack or meal as well as for general hygiene. There are no metal brackets or wires. Office visits for adjustments throughout the treatment program are fast, easy and painless. The thermoplastic aligners are virtually invisible. Over four million patients have been treated with Invisalign, and there is a special Invisalign system for teens.

Because Invisalign is computer mapped, there's sometimes the idea that anybody can install Invisalign and that all practitioners using Invisalign are the same. I have an important warning about this: during each stage of the complete treatment, only certain teeth are allowed to move. Which teeth move in what order, and the amount of time (days/weeks) needed for each successive set of aligners differs for each patient. *This* is what you rely on an expert orthodontist specializing in pediatric and juvenile care to decide. At the start, we determine whether your son or daughter is a good candidate for the

Invisalign approach, or if they would be better served with different braces. You have to rely on *somebody* to tell you. I promise you, there are kids who've been hurried to Invisalign who were not good candidates for it.

Invisalign Teen

Much like the standard adult version, the Invisalign Teen System lets you do it the modern, hygienic way. Your new smile is created with the most innovative technology—a series of clear aligners that are custom-fit to your teeth.

The first thing you should know is that an average treatment takes about a year. Plus, your treatment can begin even if you don't have all of your permanent teeth. Invisalign Teen was designed to meet your needs.

Invisalign Teen aligners will snap on your child's teeth easily. They are comfortable and practically invisible. Invisalign Teen allows for permanent teeth to grow gently while continuously moving teeth in small increments. Aligners are worn for about two weeks and then swapped for a new pair.

Invisalign Teen aligners have a "Blue Dot Wear Indicator," designed to show an estimation of wear time. The dot is designed to fade until it's clear over a two-week period if you wear your aligners properly (meaning for twenty to twenty-two hours every day).

Invisalign Teen is designed to custom-fit to your child's teeth and go with his or her lifestyle. During your treatment, your child can keep smiling, playing sports, eating what he or she wants, and brushing and flossing normally because the aligners are removable. Plus, unlike traditional braces, the aligners are made of smooth plastic and move teeth gradually.

The aligners are replaceable if lost. That's right; you get up to six free individual aligners.

After your child's Invisalign Teen treatment, you may find his or her self-confidence boosted by their new smile and the change in their appearance. Some people even feel that way during the treatment. As you know, smiling has many benefits. It can help your child make a strong impression in lots of different social situations—at school, at work, or at a party.

Invisalign Teen really works. It helps correct a broad range of dental and orthodontic issues. You can get a confident smile without metal bands, brackets, or wires. It works on many kinds of conditions, including overly crowded or widely spaced teeth, crossbites, overbites, and underbites.

We've used Invisalign to successfully transform the smiles of many patients, but we do not prescribe it to everybody. The ultimate success of Invisalign depends on two things. First, the expertise of the orthodontist in selecting the "right" types of cases and planning the treatment. Second, it's on the patient, who has to wear the aligners for twenty to twenty-four hours a day. After all, *popularity* should not govern medical care!

Trustworthy, Objective Advice

Our office is *not* "in the pocket of" or obligated to any of these providers of different braces products and technologies. We select and recommend what we believe is *the* most appropriate and beneficial choice for your child. We are happy to discuss the pros and cons of different ones, if your child has heart set on, say, Invisalign, because that's what a friend has, or based on information you've obtained.

Candidly, these manufacturers vary in price to the orthodontist (or dentist) based on volume purchase benchmarks, incentivizing concentration of as much use as possible to one product. Awards are given out to the highest volume buyers and users. It's borderline unseemly. It introduces temptation into the diagnostic and prescriptive process, and I never let us bow to such incentives and temptations. The number-one rule here is: what is absolutely best for the patient?

Call us at **352-371-3200** or go to **MartinKidsDental.com** to schedule your own Customized Smile Analysis.

Chapter Eleven

How Difficult Is Living with Braces

REMEMBER, THIS ISN'T 1982. Or 1992. Today's braces aren't anything like yours if you had them decades ago. Today's orthodontic care is far more advanced, more sophisticated, and more patient-centered than any prior generation has experienced. If you had traditional metal braces twenty years or so ago, you experienced medieval torture. The dungeon is gone too, replaced by ultra-modern, comfortable, and patient-friendly offices. Out of the dark, into the light!

Living with braces is *not* going to be anywhere near as difficult as you might imagine.

Let's look at a few specific concerns.

Brushing and Hygiene

Modern braces, whether they're metal, flexible, or "invisible," are all actually made to fit the individual and facilitate easy, painless, thorough brushing. This means your child brushes pretty much the same as he would if he didn't have braces.

Here are some simple tips you can share with your child for the best results when brushing with braces on:

- Brush your teeth with a medium nylon toothbrush after you eat and before bed (no electric toothbrushes).[2]

- Brush, rinse, and look; if you find any areas that are not clean, brush them again.

- Brush your gums as you brush your teeth (massage and stimulate).

- Take extra care in the area between the gums and the braces because food caught and left there can cause swollen gums, cavities, discomfort, and permanent teeth stains.

- If no toothpaste is available, brush without.

- If you are unable to brush, rinse your mouth vigorously with water.

- Replace your old toothbrush when it gets worn out.

- It's absolutely essential you continue regular visits to your family dentist for checkups and cleanings throughout your orthodontic treatment!

---

2   At my office, you'll be provided with a home kit including the best toothbrush, toothpaste, and rinse.

Depending on the age of your child, you, the parent, may need to supervise the first few brushings with the braces in place. You should *not* have a whining, resistant, difficult child on your hands because of any of this. It should be painless, simple, and routine.

Forbidden Foods Your Child Must Avoid

After your child's orthodontic appliance/braces have been placed, the teeth are usually "tender" and sensitive for as few as three to as many as ten days: a *short* time. During these few days, softer foods are recommended: soups, macaroni, spaghetti, eggs, fish, Jell-O, yogurt. As needed, Tylenol or Advil are adequate in relieving any discomfort, taken an hour or so before eating.[3] Warm saltwater rinses can be helpful. We also provide a "soft white wax," a safe topical that eases gum discomfort.

For the entire duration of the braces being in place, I'd advise you to stay away from hard and sticky foods that can damage braces and may lengthen the time they have to be worn or even require extra office visits. Sugar-rich foods can make hygiene harder and cause calculus build-up and cavities. You're probably already monitoring and limiting your child's intake of such foods, so there's really nothing new under the sun here. But, for the record, here are the "featured items" that should be avoided during orthodontic treatment and wearing of braces:

---

3   Prescription pain pills with dangerous side effects are not needed. Any ortho-dontist or dentist easily prescribing such drugs is not to be trusted. As you are no doubt aware from the news, opioid addiction is rampant. Pain drugs are, contrary to early assertions by their manufacturers, proving to be extremely addictive for many people after nominal and legitimate use. I can't emphasize enough—we practice truly pain-free orthodontics.

1. **Rock-hard foods**: ice (don't chew ice!), nuts, popcorn (has hard kernels inside), peanut brittle, rock candy, whole apples and carrots (unless cut into bite sized pieces), corn on the cob, hard pretzels, hard rolls, hard taco shells.

2. **Extra-sticky foods**: Jolly Ranchers or Starbursts or similar candies, bubble gum, taffy, and sticky Cinnabon rolls.

3. **Very chewy foods**: pizza crust, beef jerky, gummy bears. Note: no chewing on pencils or pens.

4. **Super sugary foods and drinks**: soda pop with sugar, ice cream, most cookies, and cake. Yes, this is the worst of the forbidden foods. Some kids will give you a tough time. But there are sugar-free versions of all these kinds of foods, to be made, baked, or store-bought.

We will speak about this with your son or daughter and give them a printed list, but *you* will have to reinforce, monitor, and provide some substitute foods to prevent mutiny or months of sulking. Most kids get it, though. When they understand how short or long the number of weeks of wearing braces will turn out to be, how comfortable or uncomfortable wearing them is, how maintaining hygiene while wearing them is, and how their results are linked to them staying away from the short list of harmful foods, they are pretty responsible about it. Most parents who are initially really worried about this tell us later it wasn't the horror show they'd imagined.

Emergencies, Injuries, Travel, and Time Away from Home

Many "emergencies" actually aren't and can be easily and safely remedied at home. You are provided with a "What to Do in Case of the Five Common Emergencies" printed card, and you can always access the same information at our web site 24/7/365.

Common emergencies include the breaking of some part of the braces, eating something particularly damaging—even a McDonalds bun full of sesame seeds might feel like an emergency, or, early, a feeling of discomfort that worries something serious might be wrong. These are the sort of things addressed in the "What to Do" instructions.

If you do run up against an emergency that isn't easily managed with these instructions or if you can't wait for regular office hours, we have a special phone number to call that routes to a knowledgeable staff member directly and who will return your call within sixty minutes or less. You are never left out to dry.

If your family or son or daughter are away from home and, say, they chomp down on a piece of toffee and break a piece of their braces, there is *always* a remedy. You are *not* going to cut your vacation short and rush to the airport! Again, often a remedy provided by our instructions can meet the urgent need until everybody gets back home. I also belong to a network of orthodontists with offices throughout the United States, which we can utilize in *the extremely rare instance* when getting to an orthodontist immediately is vital.

Here is just how good the appliances themselves and our management of orthodontic treatment has gotten. In 2016 to 2017:

- Ninety-eight percent of patients required *no* extra office visits for repairs, adjustments, care, or emergencies beyond their regularly scheduled office visits per their treatment plan.

- Eighty-five percent of patients called with questions, worries, or emergencies that were handled simply by advice and home remedy and/or waited without harm until the next regularly scheduled visit.

- Only 2 percent of patients had some problem or emergency requiring an extra, unscheduled office visit or express delivery of a temporary "patch" or solution to braces broken by sports, play, or other injury.

Sports

Speaking of injuries, the question of sports versus braces worries kids and parents alike. These days, kids are *very* active in organized and school sports, some starting one as another's season is ending. You know this; you are coordinating the schedules and working as their unpaid chauffeur.

Good news: for every sport and every level of play, there is either an inexpensive off-the-shelf mouth guard or a slightly costlier, custom-fit mouth guard to provide an extra, suitable level of dental protection and to protect the braces themselves. In some sports, additional face masks or other equipment normally treated as an option can be added and used during the time period of the orthodontic treatment. Ask us for guidance for your child and their sport(s). Some mouth guards even come with insurance against dental injury, covering financial costs.

We have thought this through! For example, research reported in *Clinics in Sports Medicine*—from the Department of Neurology at Boston University School of Medicine—examined uses of different kinds of mouth guards and the rate of sports-related concussions. There was no significant difference in concussion risks found tied to different types of mouth guards. We can select the best one for your child, their sport, and the level of play and, if a factor, your budget with no worry about one choice instead of another affecting risk of concussion.

This, by the way, is typical of a good orthodontic specialist: attention to *every* detail. They should have a good knowledge of every ramification of wearing braces, clinical and technological advancements, and every patient or parent need. To be blunt, it's a practical impossibility for a general dentist to give the braces work he does on the side anywhere near this same level of all-in focus.

By the way, there are collegiate and pro athletes—even NFL players—getting orthodontic treatment and even wearing braces. If they can, your child can! You do *not* need the drama of stopping your child from playing the sports they're committed to because of their orthodontic treatment. Oh, and we even guarantee your office visits will not cause you to miss work or business responsibilities, nor cause your child to miss school or organized sports.

See, this *isn't* going to be difficult!

Tips for Helping Your Child Adjust to a Life with Braces

- **All the cool kids are doing it (or soon will be):** Braces are a very popular appliance during the middle school and high school years. Rather than focus on how he or she feels wearing braces, encourage your child to begin actively looking for other kids who are wearing braces. Chances are, they'll find lots more than they ever imagined!

- **Even famous people do it:** Gwen Stefani. Prince Harry. Drew Barrymore. Tom Cruise. Dakota Fanning. Danny Glover. The list of famous people who've worn braces—many of them as adults—could fill half this book. Share with your child how even the most famous people in the spotlight sometimes need a little help through braces.

- **Fast forward:** Many orthodontists provide a "before and after" consultant's session, much like a plastic surgeon. Digital pictures are often used to portray what the child's teeth might look like once the braces have been removed. Have your child focus on the "after" when he or she gets down about the "before" shots!

- **Be prepared:** Finally, create a "master list" of things your child likes to do, things that make them feel special, confident, brave, calm, relaxed, or excited. If you notice them feeling down, consult your list and make plans to do something special in the near future to boost their confidence level back to where you know it belongs!

Call us at **352-371-3200** or go to **MartinKidsDental.com** to schedule your own Customized Smile Analysis.

Chapter Twelve

Life After Braces: Retainers

SO, YOUR CHILD'S BRACES are off and they're ready to live a life full of confidence and good oral health. They may think, *I'm free! I'm free!* Well, not quite yet.

The selection of the right braces, the expert orthodontist, and the compliant wearing of the braces gets us about three-fourths of the way to where we want to be: a well-aligned, as-perfect-as-possible, healthy smile for life.

But after braces, there are retainers.

While many patients are understandably eager to be done with braces once they come off, the fact is, retainers do as much work—if not more—than the braces themselves. Straight teeth in proper alignment have to stay that way, and for that, retainers are a big help.

When the braces are removed, teeth can still shift if not helped through a period of adjustment to settle in. Retainers gently but purposefully remind the teeth to stay straight during this adjustment period. It's advised that nearly all patients who've gone through the time, work, and expense of braces will want to use fixed or removable retainers for months or years or even for life. Some dentists doing braces won't tell you this, but I will. Years ago, clinicians believed that once teeth were straightened by braces, they would simply stay that way forever. New science says otherwise. In fact, teeth position shifting as we age is to be expected. Teeth naturally shift to the middle and crowd. So, retainers are actually extremely important in maintaining the new smile from braces. Any claims otherwise, by some "brand" of braces or any doctor, are flat-out false.

Retainers can play a role in:

- closing any gaps that may remain in the bite

- correcting any speech problems—sometimes occurring with a new bite or jaw position

- tongue thrust—where the tongue slips under the teeth while talking

- bruxism—grinding teeth while sleeping

As you can see, there's a lot more to this than just "installing and removing braces."

In post-braces monitoring and checkups, I tend to decide on the best kind of retainer for your child before the removal of the braces. Growth of the jaw following treatment (yes, the jaw is still growing in adolescents, to age eighteen or so), stabilization of the gums and bone tissues, pressures from lips and tongue, and other factors tell me what type of retainer should be worn and for how long. Retainers are made out of rubber, plastic, and sometimes, still, metal. They are custom made and fit as part of the complete orthodontic treatment. However, after the initial orthodontic exam, at the same time the best braces are being selected, it's usually possible, with a good degree of certainty, to predict the type of retainer(s) your child is going to need, and I'm happy to share that information with you at that time.

Some retainers are invisible or nearly invisible. There are clear plastic retainers. A *fixed* retainer is placed on the inside/back surfaces of the lower front teeth. A fixed retainer may be used until lower jaw growth is complete and then no longer needed. When your child hears "retainer" he will most likely picture a *removable* retainer. These make hygiene easy, are easily removed and cleaned daily, and can be removed for a sports activity. There are even "fashion retainers" now—popular with kids of different ages—in school colors, and some even with pictures on them! This is an important part of braces aftercare and part of the complete orthodontic treatment program personalized for your child.

Bottom line: think of retainers like going to the fitness center. If you walked out of the gym after two years with your beautiful, new body and said "I never have to workout again," you know that muscle would change if not stimulated. Similarly, as we age, the muscular forces on the teeth are constantly changing, so to keep the muscles engaged and the teeth in position, my advice is to wear a retainer as long as you want them to remain in their beautiful, new positions.

Call us at **352-371-3200** or go to **MartinKidsDental.com** to schedule your own Customized Smile Analysis.

Chapter Thirteen

Let's Celebrate!

HAVING TO WEAR BRACES can last for six months to two years or more in certain cases. During the time your child has them, they may have moved from child to preteen or preteen to teen, at times feeling embarrassed by having them, and possibly missing out on some things. They probably gave up favorite foods and snacks. They at least had to be super-conscious of what they ate and didn't eat. It's been a long time since they could sink their teeth into an apple!

You endured whatever complaining there was. You traded time to the office visits. You dealt with the "uh-oh!" and the "now what did you do?" emergencies if there were any. And, of course, you paid the bill.

We like to see our patients celebrate getting their braces off. There are so many ways your child can celebrate, everything from writing a journal about their experience to recording a video that shares their experience and shows their new look.

Here are a few options your child may want to consider:

- **Throw a party**. Throwing a "braces are off" party is a great way to celebrate. They can invite their friends over, put out the foods that they've been longing for, and they can enjoy showing off those new straight teeth. Their friends will love being able to take part in the celebration.

- **Plan a photo shoot**. Your child deserves to show the world their new beautiful smile! Plan a photo shoot, so they can be one-on-one with a photographer and put their best smile forward. They'll get some great shots and can show all their friends on social media their new look.

- **Chew some gum**. Your child might have wanted to have gum for the longest time. Although it's not the best habit, they can take an afternoon to chew some gum and feel guilt and worry free. Chew to your heart's content!

- **Go caramel**. Now is the time your child can sink their teeth into something like a caramel apple. No more avoiding the caramel and cutting the apple into bite-sized pieces. Nope, they can actually eat a full caramel apple, right off the stick! They can get one at the mall or a carnival or even make one themselves. Either way, they'll love being able to bite into that sticky gooey sweetness worry free!

- **Picnic in the park**. Weather permitting, a picnic in the park will make for a fun celebration. Take some of your child's favorite outdoor games, invite the friends, and have a cooler filled with icy drinks. On the grill, you can plan for things like corn on the cob that your child had to largely avoid while wearing their braces. It will make for a memorable afternoon!

- **Have a potluck dinner.** Have your child's friends and family each bring a dish people with braces have to take precaution with. This will give them the chance to learn a little more about what you went through, and it'll be fun to see what options they come up with. Ask each of the guests to write down a comment about your child with or without her braces. Your potluck will be filled with interesting dishes, laughs, and a good time!

- **Relax.** What could be better than spending a couple of hours being pampered, or perhaps a round of golf or fishing out on the lake? Not much! Take your child out—celebrate them making it through their treatment. They'll walk out feeling and looking great!

Doing some of these things, such as chewing gum, may still not be good for your child's teeth or their body overall. But doing it on a special occasion, and not making a habit out of it, won't cause any harm.

Of course, nobody can celebrate unless we *started*. There really is no time like the present.

Call us at **352-371-3200** or go to **MartinKidsDental.com** to schedule your own Customized Smile Analysis.

Chapter Fourteen

What About My Smile?

MOM, DAD, I'M NOT going to kid you: if braces and/or orthodontic treatment was advised when you were eight or ten or twelve and, for whatever reason, it didn't happen, and you now have misaligned teeth, periodontal problems because of them, a smile you often hide, and/or jaw/TMJ pain, it may *not* be an easy fix. It may *not* even be fixable with orthodontics or braces. But, often to the surprise of adults, braces—including invisible braces—can do a significant amount of good for people thirty, forty, or even fifty years old. You may still be able to go from an embarrassing smile you often hide to a beautiful smile you love! You'll also be able to enjoy better oral health, gently and gradually, over six to twelve months without having teeth pulled and without surgery. Many adults see ten years of age disappear from their faces!

The only way to know what the options are is with a complete, expert orthodontic exam.

While some offices may not actively seek adult patients, many will treat a lot of parents of patients, just like you, and a number of them come from referrals. You can arrange for your exam by speaking to any of the treatment coordinators at the office.

It's important to get your son or daughter the orthodontic care they need at the earliest time they are known to need it and for it to be the best care available. When that doesn't happen, it often comes around to really bite that person later in life!

Please don't ask them to hide their smile!

Call us at **352-371-3200** or go to **MartinKidsDental.com** to schedule your own Customized Smile Analysis.

"After years of being told I needed surgery, my results are amazing without it. I'm finally able to smile in holiday photos."

—JOHN W.

FAQ

Here is a handy resource guide of frequently asked questions and orthodontic terminology, many of which are answered throughout the book.

What might happen if your child's mouth doesn't quite "fit"?

The fact is, the sooner you straighten your child's smile, the faster it will develop as it should: straight, clean, and healthy!

Are there any celebrities who've worn braces?

Many! Gwen Stefani, Prince Harry, Drew Barrymore, Tom Cruise, Dakota Fanning, Danny Glover, and more.

Can I see what my child's straight teeth might look like before the procedure is done?

Yes! Digital pictures are often used to portray what the child's teeth might look like once the braces have been removed.

Will I be able to afford my child's braces?

Not only are most orthodontic procedures cheaper than ever, but insurance, payment plans, and a variety of other financing options make braces more affordable than they've ever been.

Will getting braces be painful for my child?

Not anymore! Modern technology—and choosing the right orthodontist—can ensure that your child enjoys a pain-free orthodontic experience.

How much school will my child miss because of braces?

Not much, actually. After initial visits and, barring the actual procedure itself, most visits and/or adjustments are routine and can take anywhere from fifteen to forty-five minutes.

Is it really such a big deal if my child has crooked teeth?

Unfortunately, yes. Eroding, crooked, or unaligned smiles can take time to happen, but the time to act is now. Orthodontic irregularities don't just heal on their own or "go away" if you ignore them.

What are some of the warning signs that my child might need to go to the orthodontist?

There are many, but here are a few of the most common: early or late loss of teeth, protruding teeth, grinding or clenching of teeth, and speech difficulty.

What kind of "side effects" are
caused by crooked teeth?

Some of the more frequent ones I see include headaches, tooth-aches, mouth breathing, chipped or worn down teeth, snoring, and drooling.

What makes an orthodontist more
qualified than a dentist?

Orthodontists are *dental specialists* who have completed two to three years of additional education beyond dental school to learn the proper way to align teeth and jaws.

Why should I choose a specialist for
my child's orthodontic care?

Unique treatment requirements and otherwise difficult bite problems are common, everyday scenarios for your orthodontist. In the interest of receiving the most efficient and effective orthodontic treatment possible, choose an orthodontic specialist.

How do I know if my doctor is an orthodontist?

Only orthodontists can belong to the American Association of Orthodontists (AAO).

What is a treatment coordinator?

During your initial consultation(s), you will usually be assigned a patient contact person—we call this person a "treatment coordinator" in our office—with whom you will schedule appointments, confer with rescheduling, and of course, answer any and all questions you may have.

Why are follow-up visits important?

These are wonderful opportunities to either a) ask questions you may have missed the first time, or b) get further details from your orthodontist him- or herself.

Why is early treatment so important?

Age three is the earliest time your orthodontist can determine future jaw and tooth alignment. That's because, at the age of three, your child's upper and lower jaws are developing a pattern of growth. Jaw growth sets the stage for future tooth position and serious problems can develop if the jaws are growing poorly.

Is there such a thing as a child being too old for braces?

Actually, there is. Case in point: waiting to take your child to the orthodontist until they are twelve or thirteen can be very risky. Almost all facial growth is complete by the time a child is twelve years old.

What if I don't believe in early orthodontics?

Well, you're entitled to your opinion, but this is like saying you don't believe in the sun. You can hide from it, pretend it's not there, or refuse to acknowledge it, but the simple fact remains. If you're not aware of the potential risks, you can get burnt.

Will my child actually need braces at five?

Probably not. While I inform parents their child needs an initial exam at age four, I also mention that most children *will not need braces until eleven to thirteen years of age.* Early orthodontic treatment in our office rarely involves placing braces on teeth. We focus on development of the jaws and eliminating poor oral habits that cause crooked teeth.

What is a crossbite?

When the upper and lower jaws grow at different rates, or even when the lower jaw grows disproportionately with the upper jaw, something known as a "crossbite" can occur. Usually it ocurs because of mouth breathing and the poor oral habits that stem from it.

Where should I start to look for treatment if I'm concerned about my child's jaw development?

If you suspect your child might have a crossbite or other issues, contact an orthodontic specialist. Often general dentists don't have the advanced training to recognize early developmental problems.

Why should I address a crossbite?

Crossbites can lead to pain, discomfort, and lack of confidence as your child begins to feel insecure or even ostracized because of this very treatable, very normal series of jaw and teeth developments. Kids have crossbites because the jaws are too narrow. So, you can be sure the permanent teeth will not have adequate space to come in straight.

What is Invisalign?

The Invisalign or Clear Aligner system is the virtually invisible way to straighten your teeth and achieve the dazzling smile you've always dreamed of. Using advanced 3-D computer-imaging technology, Invisalign depicts your complete treatment plan, from the initial position of your teeth to the final desired position.

What are the primary benefits of Invisalign?

Like the word that inspired them, Invisalign aligners are practically clear and as close to "invisible" as one can get. No one may even notice you're wearing these virtually invisible braces, making Invisalign a seamless fit with your lifestyle and day-to-day interactions with others.

How do I get started with Invisalign?

It's simple: just make an appointment with your local orthodontist for an initial consultation. Most doctors will offer a free initial consultation to see if you are a good candidate for Invisalign.

How will Invisalign effectively move my teeth?

Aligners are the foundation for, and work in unison with, the Invisalign system. Like brackets and arch wires are to braces, Invisalign aligners move teeth by using the appropriate placement of controlled force on your child's teeth.

How many patients are being treated with Invisalign?

More than one million patients worldwide have been treated with Invisalign. The number of Invisalign smiles grows daily.

Is Invisalign appropriate for my child?

Yes, especially because Invisalign now has a system designed specifically for teens!

How does Invisalign Teen work?

Aligners snap on your teeth easily. They are comfortable and practically invisible. Invisalign Teen allows permanent teeth to grow and gently and continuously moves your teeth in small increments. Aligners are worn for about two weeks, then you swap them for a new pair.

Why are metal braces still so popular?

Metal braces are very strong and can withstand most types of treatment. Today's metal braces are smaller, sleeker, and more polished than ever before.

Are so-called "clear braces" effective?

Ceramic braces are very strong and generally do not stain. Adults like to choose ceramic braces because they "blend in" with the teeth and are less noticeable than metal. These are the types of braces actor Tom Cruise had.

Are clear braces appropriate for adults?

Absolutely! Adults of all ages can enjoy the same cosmetic and health benefits of properly aligned teeth with clear braces.

What are some of my payment options in addition to insurance?

One way many patients pay for their procedures is by utilizing the benefits of what is known as "flex spending," where their employer matches their spending commitment.

What if my child has a "braces emergency" before or after office hours?

If you are experiencing an orthodontic emergency that can't wait for regular office hours, most orthodontic offices have a special number to call, either before, during, or after business hours. If this information isn't given to you readily, ask how your doctor's office handles emergencies. I give every patient my personal cell phone number as I would if they were a family member I was treating.

Can a salt water rinse help deal with irritation caused by braces?

Absolutely; warm saltwater rinses soothe the cheek lining, which can get aggravated by your child's braces.

How do I make a salt water rinse?

To make a salt water rinse, mix half a teaspoon of table salt in one cup of warm water. Stir until the salt is completely dissolved. Gently swish about a fourth of the cup in your mouth for thirty seconds. Make sure you force the water over the areas that feel sore. Then spit the water into the sink. Repeat until the entire cup is gone.

What if my child plays sports and needs a mouth guard?

The best advice for patients or parents looking for a mouth guard can be obtained from your pediatrician, dentist, children's dentist, orthodontist or oral surgeon. All of these specialists are uniquely trained to offer customized advice in order to help you prevent a sports-related dental or facial injury.

What about brushing with braces?

Here are some simple tips you can share with your child for the best results when brushing with braces on:

- Brush your teeth with a medium nylon toothbrush after you eat and before bed.

- Brush, rinse, and look; if you find any areas that are not clean, brush them again.

- Brush your gums as you brush your teeth (massage and stimulate).

- If no toothpaste is available, brush without.

- If you are unable to brush, rinse your mouth vigorously with water.

- Replace your old toothbrush when it gets worn out.

- It is absolutely essential that you continue regular visits to your family dentist for checkups and cleanings throughout your orthodontic treatment!

What type of foods should my child avoid while wearing braces?

There are four main types of food your child should avoid while wearing braces: (1) **hard foods**, like ice, popcorn, peanut brittle, rock candy, and corn on the cob, (2) **sticky foods**, like caramels, bubble gum, taffy, and suckers, (3) **chewy foods**, like pizza crust, crusty breads, beef jerky, and gummy bears, and (4) **sugary foods and drinks**, like cake, ice cream, cookies, pie, candy, and soda pop.

Why are retainers so important?

As we age, teeth naturally shift to the middle and crowd. Combined with late growth of the lower jaw, shifting of the teeth is expected following orthodontic treatment. Therefore, retainers are extremely important in the maintenance of your new smile following orthodontic treatment.

Resources

Before or after your consultation, you may want more information for yourself or your son or daughter. The following websites provide valuable insight to help you make the right decision for your child.

Braces.org is the "all about braces site" of the American Association of Orthodontists. This is the official regulatory body and professional association of orthodontists, and *only* orthodontists (*not* dentists) can be members. Here you will receive accurate, up-to-date information on orthodontics.

About the Author

SPEAKER, TEACHER, AUTHOR, and orthodontic specialist Dr. Bill Martin has created over thirty thousand beautiful smiles in children and adults since founding Martin Orthodontics in 1979. If you speak to him directly, however, you'll quickly realize that this numeric description barely scratches the surface of his expertise. When asked to describe what he does, Dr. Martin replies, "I help children to breathe better, sleep better, grow better, and look better, so they can perform better at school, in sports, and socially. …Oh, and I'm an orthodontist, too."

Dr. Martin has devoted his life to the health and well-being of children, and he puts his significant scientific and medical expertise to work in this regard. In 2013, Dr. Martin founded Martin Kids Dental Health Team to provide comprehensive dental and orthodontic care for children in the Gainesville, Florida, area. Thanks to his unique expertise in childhood airway development, Dr. Martin regularly provides critical guidance and education to parents, helping them to transform their children into peak performers in school and at play.

In so doing, Dr. Martin has cultivated an outstanding reputation in the Gainesville, Florida, area for his skillful and honest approach to children's health through orthodontic and dental medicine.

Today, Dr. Martin stands as a pioneer in Airway Orthodontics, a revolutionary sub-specialty of orthodontic medicine. Airway Orthodontics follows an interdisciplinary approach to combating sleep breathing disorders, especially in children. Dr. Martin's notable expertise in Airway Orthodontics stems in part from his willingness to study and gain experience beyond the boundaries of the traditional orthodontic profession. In particular, Dr. Martin specializes in breathing disorders, sleep disorders, and over all physical and cognitive growth in children.

A firm believer in continuing education, Dr. Martin regularly supplements his medical knowledge both in and beyond the field of orthodontics. He achieves this through numerous professional memberships, conferences, and continuing medical education courses.

Dr. Martin is a current member of the American Association of Orthodontists, the Southern Association of Orthodontists, the Florida Association of Orthodontists, the American Dental Association, the Florida Dental Association, the Alachua County Dental Society, the American Academy of Pediatric Dentistry, the American Association of Sleep Medicine, and the American Association of Dental Sleep Medicine.

THE
NEXT
STEP

Your Customized Smile Analysis

When you are ready, I urge you to schedule your Customized Smile Analysis, complete with a complimentary consultation, safe, digital x-rays (a $350 value) an exam, and a report provided to you and your son or daughter—all without cost or obligation.

Call us at **352-371-3200** or go to **MartinKidsDental.com**.

Printed in the USA
CPSIA information can be obtained
at www.ICGtesting.com
JSHW012037140824
68134JS00033B/3114

9 781599 329338